plastic surgery of the female breast

R.C.A. WEATHERLEY-WHITE, M.D., F.A.C.S.

Associate Clinical Professor of Surgery (Plastic),
University of Colorado Medical Center,
Denver, Colorado

drawings by John Parker
operative photography by Hasi Vogel

plastic surgery of the female breast

HARPER & ROW, PUBLISHERS

HAGERSTOWN

Cambridge
New York
Philadelphia
San Francisco

London
Mexico City
São Paulo
Sydney

1817

The authors and publisher have exerted every effort to ensure that drug selection and dosage set forth in this text are in accord with current recommendations and practice at the time of publication. However, in view of ongoing research, changes in government regulations, and the constant flow of information relating to drug therapy and drug reactions, the reader is urged to check the package insert for each drug for any change in indications and dosage and for added warnings and precautions. This is particularly important when the recommended agent is a new or infrequently employed drug.

1 3 5 6 4 2

Library of Congress Cataloging in Publication Data

Weatherley-White, R C A
    Plastic surgery of the female breast.

    Includes index.
    1. Mammaplasty—Atlases. 2. Breast—Surgery—Atlases. 3. Breast —Surgery—Psychological aspects. I. Title. [DNLM: 1. Breast—Surgery—Atlases. 2. Surgery, Plastic—Atlases. 3. Breast neoplasms— Surgery—Atlases. WP17 W362p] RD539.8.W42 618.1'9 79-22187
ISBN 0-06-142630-X

*To my wife, Dorian, for her loving encouragement and
endless cups of early morning tea*

contents

contributors

DAVID M. CHARLES, M.D., F.C.S. (S.A.)
CHAPTERS 1, 6

Assistant Clinical Professor of Surgery (Plastic),
University of Colorado Medical Center,
Denver, Colorado

DENNIS M. MAHONEY, M.D., J.D.
CHAPTER 7, legal aspects

Johnson and Mahoney, P.C.
Denver, Colorado

RICHARD H. MCSHANE, M.D.
CHAPTER 6

Director and Head of the Division of Plastic Surgery,
Albany Medical College, Union University,
Albany, New York

RICHARD L. VANDENBERGH, M.D.
CHAPTER 7, psychosocial aspects

Associate Clinical Professor of Psychiatry,
University of Colorado Medical Center,
Denver, Colorado

R.C.A. WEATHERLEY-WHITE, M.D., F.A.C.S.
CHAPTERS 2, 3, 4, 5, 6

Associate Clinical Professor of Surgery (Plastic),
University of Colorado Medical Center,
Denver, Colorado

ix

foreword

What a fortuitous time for Dr. Weatherley-White to be writing upon surgery of the female breast! Fifteen years ago such a treatise would have contained only a few somewhat crude breast reductions, and mammary augmentations by free grafts of dermis, dermis-fat and de-epithelialized flaps.

Today, however, Dr. Weatherley-White is able to assemble between the covers of this book multitudinous techniques for reduction of the breast. In addition, there is the nearly 15-year-old "track record" of the successful mammary prosthesis devised by Cronin and Gerow, bringing permanency to breast augmentation. It is the breast prosthesis which has become the **sine qua non** of breast construction following ablation for carcinoma or precancerous lesions, also covered in this text.

It seems to be tacitly agreed that a surgical atlas is as good as its illustrator, and often to the artist belongs any kudos the volume may deserve. I tend to think of the contributions of such medical illustrators as Mildred Codding, Gertrude Hance, Max Broedel, Daisy Stilwell, Leonard Dank, as often as the surgeons who supplied procedures and text.

This atlas, however, is treated in a manner different from the usual, for here the photographer's print is at least as important as the artist's drawing. This lends credence to the technical ability of the author, so important to the dexterous elite of surgery.

Beyond the explicit depiction of operative techniques, Dr. Weatherley-White wisely has added a chapter on malpractice and psychiatric aspects of aesthetic surgery of the breast, important information to all who would trespass surgically into the fragile realm of body-image surgery.

Here is an atlas that for the aesthetic plastic surgeon is both useful and timely.

Richard Boies Stark, M.D.
Professor of Clinical Surgery,
Columbia University College
of Physicians and Surgeons,
New York, New York

preface

The female breast, as pointed out in the first chapter of this book, has been since time immemorial the universal symbol of womanhood, fertility, and attractive femininity. Reconstruction of a breast disfigured by disease, congenital abnormality, ablative surgery, or the inexorable effects of aging has presented an extraordinary challenge to plastic surgeons the world over. Each year a significant proportion of the plastic surgery literature is devoted to new procedures or modifications of established operations which attempt to recreate the perfect, or at least acceptable, breast.

It seemed appropriate to tie this wealth of information into a single volume for the use of the surgeon—plastic, general, or gynecologic—who may be somewhat ill-at-ease in dealing with the myriad varieties of breast deformity. A number of excellent texts (by Goldwyn, Georgiade, and others) have been published; they are significant contributions. However, there is still a need for an operative atlas which will take the less experienced surgeon, step-by-step, through the various procedures which one will be required to perform.

Reconstructive breast surgery is a subtle art, requiring the highest standards of both tissue management and aesthetic appreciation. Pitfalls lurk, and errors both of judgment and technique will be made. I have tried in this book to point out the more obvious mistakes, some of which I have made myself, and to stress the management of complications which are inevitable when one has a large series of cases.

The principal purpose of the book is, however, to illustrate the operative techniques used in plastic surgery of the breast. These are arranged in chapters according to their reasonably obvious categories. Drawings are invaluable to illustrate historic procedures and to demonstrate the fine details of planning and execution of contemporary operations. In this book the magnificent art work of Mr. John Parker fulfills these needs.

Yet drawings, however accurate, are always a little **too** perfect to capture the subtle variations of tissue which in "real life" present themselves to the surgeon at the operating table. Only by means of photographs of the actual, unsimplified, and unidealized operative situation can the details of the technique be shown to the surgeon faced with practical decisions.

Generally, operative photographs taken during a procedure are messy, unclear, and cluttered with irrelevant detail. I have been fortunate enough to acquire the services of a highly talented photographer, Ms. Hasi Vogel, who has brought to surgical photography the same clarity and discipline which have won her acclaim in the fields of architectural and sculptural photography. The operative sequences, in my opinion, distinguish this atlas from its illustrious predecessors. Each procedure is carried through from planning to final result, and shows in clear detail the steps necessary to achieve this result.

Each clinical chapter is arranged in the same sequence—historical background, contemporary procedures, management of complications, and the author's choice of technique. If, in the last section, I have unconsciously plagiarized the work of others, I crave indulgence. Often an idea will germinate (prompted by suggestions or half-remembered presentations of merit), develop in the author's mind, become modified, improved (sometimes), until it emerges full-fledged as an "original" act of creation. Such is always the way of those of us who strive, consciously or unconsciously, to improve our performance.

In addition to those who have inadvertently lent their influence to this book, I would like to express appreciation to my official collaborators, Dr. David M. Charles, Dr. Richard L. VandenBergh, Dr. Dennis M. Mahoney, and Dr. Richard H. McShane, for their expert contributions. Each has added an invaluable dimension to the scope of the volume.

A surgeon of middling experience has, inevitably, many influences on his or her professional life. In my case, Dr. Francis Moore, Mosley Professor of Surgery at the Peter Bent Brigham Hospital, first sowed the seeds of interest in the field of surgery to an enthusiastic but vaguely directed medical student. My principal plastic surgery teachers were Dr. Richard B. Stark, former Chief of Plastic Surgery at St. Luke's Hospital in New York City, and the late C.R. McLaughlin, F.R.C.S.(E.), consultant at the Queen Victoria Hospital, East Grinstead, in the U.K. I am sure that both were driven to distraction by a constant barrage of questions, but each was generous and tolerant, and patiently instilled the principles of judgment and technique into their trainee.

I would like to express my gratitude to my senior colleagues in general surgery, Dr. Henry Swan, Dr. William Waddell, Dr. Tom Starzl, and Dr. Ben Eiseman, who all, in different ways, encouraged my fledgling efforts to develop the field of plastic surgery in Colorado, and lent their support to the writing of this book.

Finally, my heartfelt thanks to my patients, who have had the trust and confidence which allowed me to develop the techniques described in the forthcoming pages.

R.C.A. W-W.

plastic surgery of the female breast

1

anatomy of the breast

DAVID M. CHARLES

The female breast is a universal symbol of womanhood that can be traced in mythology and art from the earliest cave drawings, through every major epoch and era to modern times, and even to the centerfolds of popular magazines. The milk-secreting function of the breast which is required for suckling the young is a principal characteristic of the class of animals, the Mammalia, to which the species **Homo sapiens** belongs. The breast is identical in males and females, boys and girls, and differs only in quantitative degrees in the mature female.

Transcending its nurturing function, the breast has assumed vast psychosexual importance, and the loss of a breast in the female often has the psychological impact that castration has in the male.[26] The breast is the classical link between the mother and child and is the first means by which the child will investigate the world around him. It imparts warmth, pleasure, and comfort to the infant and cements the bond between mother and child.

Men have always been intrigued by the breast; initially it is an important part of sexual exploration, and often it is the first site of physical contact at the start of intimacy. Women in general respond to social pressures regarding the breast with a deep desire to conform to the desired size and shape of the idealized breast. The flat-chested flappers of the 1920s and the unisex fashion modes of the 1960s were but short-lived periods of haute couture.

We are truly a **mammarized** society.

EMBRYOLOGY

The human breast develops in the pectoral portion of the "milk line," which is an ectodermal ridge extending from the axilla down the chest and the abdomen to the vulva and the medial aspects of the upper thighs.[1]

The milk line develops during the sixth week of intrauterine life, and by the ninth week only the pectoral portion remains. The nipple bud begins as a mass of basal cells which heap up and which are later invaded by squamous cells that will grow downward to form the mammary ducts (Fig. 1-1). From this epithelial ridge of the nipple bud, a total of from 15 to 20 solid cords will grow down into the underlying mesenchymal tissue.

The prepubertal mammary gland consists of simple epithelial-lined ducts. These later bud out to form the alveoli which will eventually produce milk.

Under normal circumstances, a pair of breasts will develop in the pectoral region. Occasionally accessory nipples, sometimes accompanied by secretory glandular tissue, will develop in ectopic sites along this mammary line (Fig. 1-2). Ectopic breast tissue may enlarge during pregnancy[22] and is subject to all the diseases to which normal breast tissue is liable.[32] Breast carcinoma can occur in an ectopic site and can be difficult to diagnose, usually being first recognized in the pathologic examination of a biopsy specimen of a lump situated along the milk line.[29]

TOPOGRAPHY OF THE BREAST

The breast is situated on the anterolateral aspect of the chest, extending from the sternum to the anterior axillary line and from the second to the sixth ribs (Fig. 1-3). The female breast is roughly hemispherical with a circular outline, a flattened posterior aspect, and a convex subcutaneous surface. It has a lateral extension, the axillary tail (of Spence), which runs upward and laterally through a defect in the axillary fascia (Lange's foramen) to lie within the axilla itself.

MUSCULAR RELATIONSHIPS OF THE BREAST

About two-thirds of the breast is situated on the pectoralis major muscle. The pectoralis minor muscle lies completely behind the pectoralis major

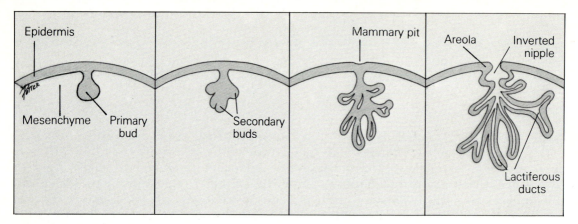

FIG. 1–1.

The evolution of the nipple. **A.** Thickening of epidermis with formation of primary bud which grows into mesenchyme. **B.** Formation of solid secondary buds. **C.** Formation of mammary pit and vacuolation of buds to form epithelial-lined ducts. **D.** Lactiferous ducts proliferate. Areola is formed. Nipple is inverted initially.

muscle. The inferolateral part of the breast lies on the lower digitations of the serratus anterior and the inferomedial part on the external oblique and rectus abdominis muscles. These muscles are covered by the deep fascia and the breast is attached to this fascia by loose connective tissue which forms the potential retromammary space.

BREAST MEASUREMENTS AND AESTHETIC CONCEPTS

Penn[24] attempted to establish standards of normality in the size and shape of the breast. The measurements of 20 models with aesthetically perfect breasts indicated that there were negligible variations between certain key landmarks, these measurements being surprisingly independent of the women's height and weight. On the average, the distance from the suprasternal notch to the nipple forms an equilateral triangle, with an internipple distance of approximately 21 cm. Spratt[30] states that the average cephalocaudal dimension is 10 to 12 cm. The nonlactating breast weighs 150 to 200 g.

The breast is soft because its contained fat is in a semifluid state, and the position of the body in relation to the pull of gravity affects the shape of the

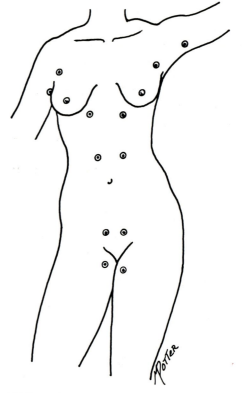

FIG. 1–2.

Sites of supernumerary nipples along "milk line." Ectopic nipple, areola, or breast tissue can develop from the groin to the axilla and upper inner arm. They can lactate or undergo malignant change.

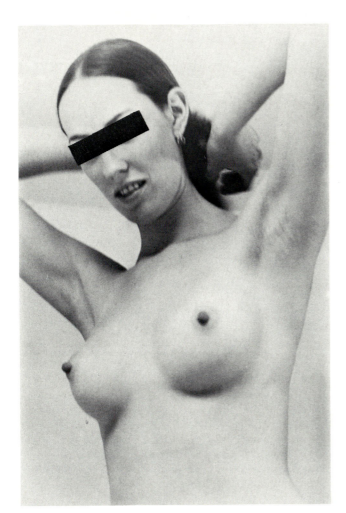

FIG. 1–3.
The topography of the mature female breast. The breast is situated on the anterolateral aspect of the chest. The contained fat is in a semifluid state and its position and shape are affected by gravity.

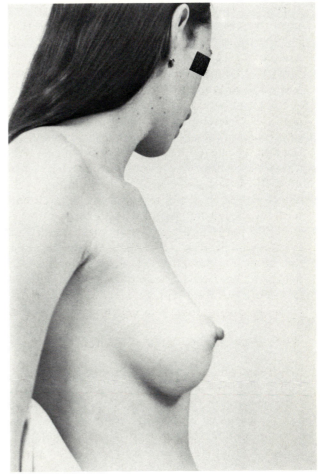

FIG. 1–4.
The profile of the female breast. The classic fluid curves of the breast in the upright position.

breast. In a supine position, the breasts tend to flatten out and flow over the lateral side of the chest toward the axilla. In the upright position, there is a caudal flow of breast tissue which, on profile, gives it the classical fluid series of concave and convex curves (Fig. 1-4). In profile, the superior surface of the breast appears concave, whereas the inferior margin is convex. The nipple and areola project near the center of the breast as two further convex curves.

THE MAMMARY DUCT SYSTEM

The secretory portion of the breast is composed of secretory acini which cluster to make up lobules; these in turn aggregate to form the lobes of the gland. There are 15 to 20 of these lobes arranged in a radiating fashion, and they drain centripetally into lactiferous ducts. The lactiferous ducts dilate to form sinuses underneath the areola and then narrow to traverse the nipple opening by little orifices on its summit. Fat fills the interstices between the tubuloglandular structure of the breast.

Hicken[12] carefully studied the ramifications of the lactiferous ducts over the anterolateral aspect of the chest (Fig. 1-5). In 95 per cent of cases the ducts ascended into the axilla and occasionally followed the brachial plexus and axillary vessels into the apex of the axilla. In 15 per cent of cases the ducts were found in the epigastric region. Occasionally the ducts passed across the midline of the chest. Breast tissue is found in intimate contact with the dermis and penetrates the deep fascia of the chest muscles as well. Goldman and Goldwyn[8] have emphasized the incompleteness of glandular resection in subcutaneous mastectomies. Recently, Krook[14] has described the significantly different rates of breast cancer development with different mammographic parenchymal patterns.

THE FASCIA OF THE BREAST

The breast is contained entirely within the superficial fascia.[30] The parenchymatous tissue of the breast is situated within a fatty areolar layer which is continuous with Camper's fatty superficial abdominal fascia below and with the superficial cervical fascia above. On the deep aspect of the breast is a layer of denser fibrous tissue. There is a loose

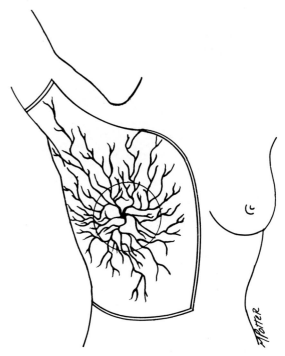

FIG. 1–5.
The extensive ramifications of the lactiferous ducts. The ducts extend onto the upper medial aspect of the arm, to the midline, and into the epigastrium. A composite drawing from mammographic studies. (After Hicken, N.F.: Mastectomy. A clinical pathologic study demonstrating why most mastectomies result in incomplete removal of the mammary gland. Arch. Surg., **40**:6, 1940)

layer of connective tissue which fills the potential retromammary space between the breast and its investing fascia and the deep fascia of the muscles of the chest wall.

The fascia covering the anterior aspect of the pectoralis major muscle is attached in the midline to the anterior aspect of the sternum and superiorly to the clavicle.[17] Laterally and inferiorly this fascia continues downward to the thorax and across the root of the axilla. It is this part which is pierced by the axillary tail of the breast. A covering is given to the axillary vessels, forming a vascular sheath. The fascia extends over the serratus anterior and is firmly attached to it. The nerve to the serratus anterior (long thoracic nerve of Bell) is closely applied to the fascia covering this muscle. Damage to this nerve results in inability to stabilize the scapula to the thorax, a condition called "winging of the scapula."

The fascia lining the deep aspect of the pectoralis major is continuous with the fascia investing the pectoralis minor. This fascia continues superiorly, splitting to enclose the subclavius muscle. That part of the fascia between the pectoralis minor and the clavicle is known as the clavipectoral fascia. It forms a dense layer protecting the underlying axillary vessels.[17] Medially, the same layer of fascia blends with the fascial covering of the muscles of the first and second intercostal spaces, and laterally, it is attached to the coracoid process. Below the pectoralis minor muscle a fascial band, known as the suspensory ligament of the axilla, continues downward and fuses with the axillary fascia. The clavipectoral fascia is pierced by the thoracoacromial artery, the cephalic vein, and the lateral pectoral nerve.

THE LIGAMENTS OF COOPER

The framework of fascial bands called the suspensory ligaments of Cooper traverse the gland, separating and supporting the lobules and attaching the skin of the breast to the underlying pectoral fascia (Fig. 1-6). Cancer of the breast involves these ligaments and causes dimpling of the skin by involvement and contracture of the ligaments of Cooper. These same bands will fix the skin to a malignancy so that the skin cannot be freely moved over it. In addition, if the tumor grows along the bands toward the pectoral fascia, it will form a fixed mass in the breast.[16] Loss of tone in these ligaments, such as following pregnancy and lactation, will result in ptosis of the breast.

THE NIPPLE AND AREOLA

The site of the nipple is variable, depending upon the position of the body and the pendulousness of the breast. Usually, it is opposite the fourth intercostal space. The nipples and areolae of women and men, girls and boys, are qualitatively identical but quantitatively different.[20]

The epidermis of the nipple and areola has long dermal papillae and an elaborate understructure of epidermal ridges (Fig. 1-7). Presumably this is to protect the nipple from excoriation and damage from the suckling infant.

The surface of the nipple and areola is glabrous and heavily pigmented due to the many melanocytes which are distributed throughout the skin, the duct system, and the sebaceous glands.

The 15 to 20 lactiferous ducts open on the apex of the nipple, and there are groups of large sebaceous glands which are found between the ducts opening onto the tip as well as the sides of the nipple and into the ducts themselves. The rich capillary circulation brings blood close to the surface of the skin of the nipple and areola, contributing to the pink color of the nipple.

There is an elaborate pattern of elastic fibers arranged parallel to the ducts and circumferentially throughout the nipple and areola. Contraction of smooth muscle reduces the surface area of the areola and results in erection of the nipple. The terminal portions of the lactiferous ducts are surrounded by bundles of smooth muscle which act as a sphincter.[7]

The nipple and areola undergo pigmentation

FIG. 1–6.
Schematic representation of the ligaments of Cooper. The ligaments suspend the 15 to 20 lobes of the breast within a matrix of fat. They are attached to the lobes, the skin, and the deep fascia.

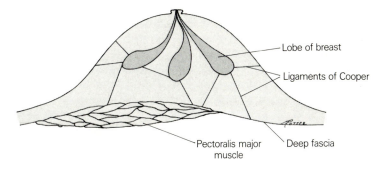

Lobe of breast

Ligaments of Cooper

Pectoralis major muscle

Deep fascia

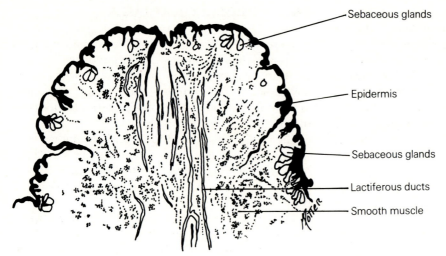

FIG. 1–7.
Cross-section of the nipple. The epidermis has long dermal papillae, is glabrous and heavily pigmented. Sebaceous glands are found near the tip and along the sides of the nipple.

changes which begin at birth with a steroid-mediated phase of melanocyte activity.[6] The second phase of activity occurs during pregnancy when the light pink to brown color darkens during the second month of the first pregnancy and never regains its pristine color. There is also evidence of progressive increase in areolar pigmentation in multiple pregnancies and after the sixth decade of life. The areola contains large sweat and sebaceous glands which usually are unassociated with hairs.

The understructure of the epidermis of the areola is not as elaborate as that of the nipple and is intermediate between the structure of the skin of the nipple (which is similar to the volar skin of the hand) and the surrounding skin of the breast (which resembles the skin of the rest of the body). There are a few hair follicles near the periphery of the areola.

Montgomery, in 1856,[1] described soft papules on the female areola which he interpreted to be sebaceous glands. There has been much debate as to the exact nature of these structures, and Giacometti[7] has referred to them as accessory mammary glands. Ackerman[1] concludes that Montgomery's opinion that the papules are composed of sebaceous glands is correct.

Montagna[20,21] has given an exhaustive account of the areolar tubercles of Montgomery. There are six to ten of these tubercles randomly distributed within the inner two-thirds of the areola. Each tubercle is composed of three to six Montgomery ducts usually associated with one or two sebaceous

glands that frequently open into one of the ducts. Montagna[21] believes that the glands of Montgomery are similar in every respect to the major ducts and glands of the breast and are an integral part of the mammary apparatus.

INNERVATION OF THE HUMAN FEMALE BREAST

Surgical anatomy of the nerve supply of the breast is important for the planning of both reduction and augmentation mammaplasty. The surgeon attempts to preserve the nerve supply in order to preserve nipple sensitivity and sensuality. The nipple is innervated principally by the anterior and lateral cutaneous branches of the fourth intercostal nerve. The third and fifth intercostal nerves participate in an overlapping fashion as well.[31] The rest of the breast is supplied by the lateral branches of the anterior cutaneous and the anterior branches of the lateral cutaneous nerves of the third and sixth intercostal nerves.

The nerves course along the anterior surface of the pectoralis major muscle close to the deep fascia before turning outward through the substance of the mammary gland to reach the nipple itself (Fig. 1-8). The supraclavicular nerves (from the cervical plexus) supply the upper part of the breast, and the intercostobrachial and the third and fourth lateral cutaneous nerves supply the axillary tail of the breast.

The skin of the breast has a fairly normal distribution of sensory nerve end-organs. On the other

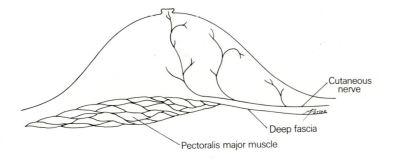

FIG. 1-8.
Schematic representation of the nerve supply of the breast and nipple. The cutaneous nerves run close to the deep fascia before turning outward toward the skin.

Cutaneous nerve

Deep fascia

Pectoralis major muscle

hand, the skin of the nipple and areola is poorly supplied with these end-organs.[18] Only the tip of the nipple has demonstrable end-organs,[19] and they are also found around the terminal portions of the lactiferous ducts and sinuses and tubercles of Montgomery, and presumably are the receptors and efferent pathway for the neurohumoral control of lactation. The neural elements of the nipple lie in the center of the nipple and follow the milk ducts to the tip of the nipple. The vellus hair roots and smooth muscle fibers are also well supplied with nerves.

Miller[18] has documented the sparsity of epidermal and papillary dermal nerve end-organs in the nipple and areola, which is probably related to the lack of superficial sensory acuity. This is contrary to the popular belief that the nipples and areola are highly sensitive erogenous areas.

Courtiss and Goldwyn[4] measured breast sensation in a large number of patients both before and after breast surgery. They used a device that emitted a variable current producing a burning sensation when the threshold stimulus was exceeded. The result showed that the areola was the most sensitive and the nipple the least sensitive part of the breast. The skin of the breast was of intermediate sensitivity. Postoperatively, the more extensive the surgery, the greater the decrease in sensation.

THE VASCULAR ANATOMY OF THE BREAST

The surgical outcome of many breast operations is dependent upon accurate knowledge of the vascular anatomy of the breast. There still appears to be no consensus on the exact description of the blood supply of the breast. Sir Astley Cooper published his classic chronicle on the anatomy of the breast in 1840. Since then, Manchot,[15] in 1889, Kaufman,[15] in 1933, Salmon,[28] in 1939, Maliniac,[15] in 1943, and Cunningham,[5] in 1977, have provided further descriptions of the blood supply of the breast.

The breast is chiefly supplied by the subclavian artery, of which the internal thoracic (internal mammary) artery is a branch and the axillary a continuation.[5] In addition, there is a small contribution from the mammary branches of the posterior intercostal arteries which are derived from the aorta.

The Lateral Mammary Artery

The classic term for the major artery of the breast is the **lateral thoracic artery**. It has also been called the **principle external artery of the breast**. A true lateral thoracic artery varies in size and position and is frequently absent. When it is present, the lateral mammary artery runs over the axillary tail of the breast, being about 1 to 2 mm. in diameter and lying at a depth of 10 to 25 mm. in the subcutaneous fatty tissue (Fig. 1-9). It supplies the breast and ends by joining the other mammary arteries in a plexus which arborizes throughout the parenchyma of the gland and which tends to radiate and concentrate toward the nipple. The lateral mammary artery may arise as a branch of the lateral thoracic artery or directly from the axillary artery. Rarely, it may arise from the thoracoacromial artery or from the subscapular arteries.

Anterior Medial Mammary Arteries

The anterior perforating branches of the internal mammary artery pass forward through the medial end of the intercostal spaces accompanying the anterior cutaneous branches of the intercostal nerve (Fig. 1-10). They pass through spaces 1 through 4

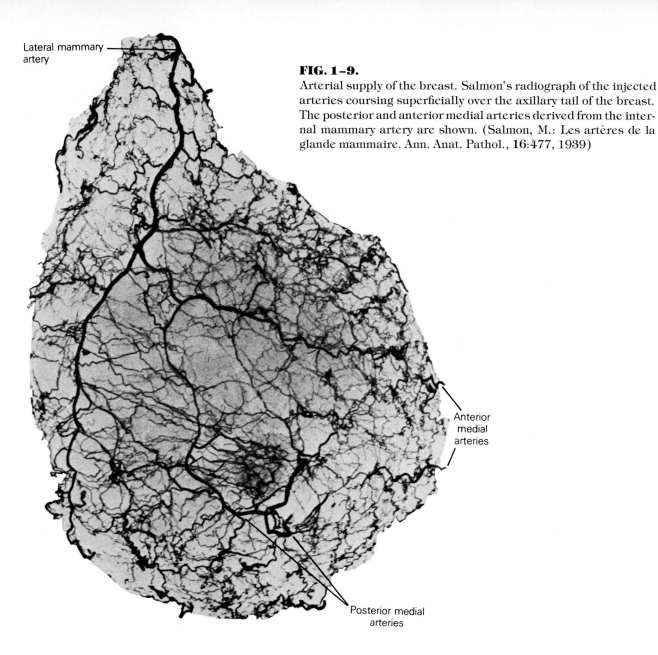

Lateral mammary artery

FIG. 1–9.

Arterial supply of the breast. Salmon's radiograph of the injected arteries coursing superficially over the axillary tail of the breast. The posterior and anterior medial arteries derived from the internal mammary artery are shown. (Salmon, M.: Les artères de la glande mammaire. Ann. Anat. Pathol., **16**:477, 1939)

Anterior medial arteries

Posterior medial arteries

and divide into a cutaneous and a mammary branch. There are usually no more than two anterior medial mammary arteries to each side. The diameter of these arteries is similar to that of the lateral mammary arteries and their depth is 5 to 15 mm. They join the plexus of arteries which ramifies throughout the breast.

Posterior Medial Mammary Arteries

These vessels are mentioned by Salmon[28] and described by Cunningham[5] (Fig. 1-11). They are branches of the internal mammary artery. They traverse the intercostal spaces perforating the pectoralis major muscle and have a tortuous course on the anterior surface of the pectoralis major running in the retromammary space. They traverse the space perforating the breast on the posterior aspect and anastomose with other branches within the breast.

Arteries of Lesser Importance

The pectoral branch of the thoracoacromial artery runs in the space between the pectoralis major and minor muscles. It traverses the pectoralis major

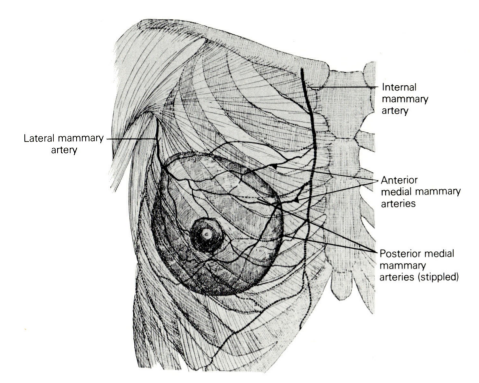

Internal mammary artery

Lateral mammary artery

Anterior medial mammary arteries

Posterior medial mammary arteries (stippled)

FIG. 1–10.
Schematic representation of the arterial supply of the breast. (Salmon, M.: les artères de la glande mammaire. Ann. Anat. Pathol., **16**:477, 1939)

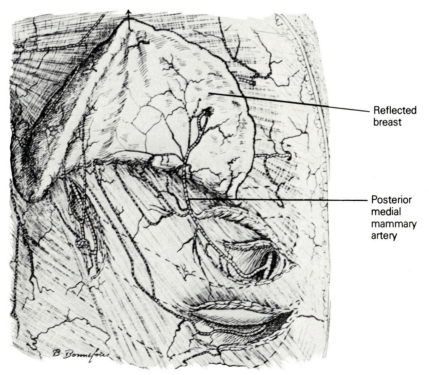

Reflected breast

Posterior medial mammary artery

FIG. 1–11.
The posterior medial mammary arteries. Salmon's diagram of the reflected breast showing these vessels originating from the internal mammary artery, then penetrating the intercostal muscles before crossing the retromammary space and entering the deep aspect of the mammary gland. (Salmon, M.: Les artères de la glande mammaire. Ann. Anat. Pathol., **16**: 477, 1939)

muscle, accompanied by veins and lymphatics, and enters the posterior surface of the breast.

Mammary branches of the posterior intercostal arteries which are derived from the aorta arise variably from the fourth and fifth posterior intercostal arteries and run in the retromammary space before passing into the breast substance.

The Arterial Plexus of Salmon

The previously described arteries break up into a plexus which communicates freely in the subcutaneous fat layer of the breast. From the superficial and deep parts of the plexuses there are branches which run toward the base of the nipple and the areola, resulting in a rich periareolar blood supply. Maliniac[15] has described three kinds of periareolar plexuses, namely, a circular type, a loop plexus, and a radial plexus. He felt this was important because he postulated that necrosis of the central portions of the breast was less likely to occur with the circular periareolar plexus which he found occurring in 70 to 74 per cent of breasts examined. The loop type, which occurred in 20 per cent, and the radial type, which occurred in 6 per cent, were more liable to central breast necrosis.

Deep to the areola the subcutaneous tissue thins out and disappears so that the areola is in close contact with the periareolar plexus of the breast.

The Venous Drainage of the Breast

The venous drainage is very variable, and the veins do not necessarily follow the arterial supply. There is also a marked asymmetry of the venous drainage. There are two systems, a superficial and a deep system (Fig. 1-12). A few veins end directly into the external jugular vein. The superficial veins of the breast can frequently be seen with the naked eye, especially when they become engorged during pregnancy. Blood drains from the superficial to the deep system and then into the internal mammary, axillary, and cephalic veins. A subareolar plexus of radiating veins drains into a periareolar vein which is polygonal in shape and appears to be the principal link between the superficial and deep venous systems.[5]

Two patterns of venous drainage have been described but their existence appears to be in doubt. A transverse pattern converges toward the sternum, whereas a longitudinal pattern drains toward the neck.

It has been implied that the vertebral venous system accounts for breast cancer metastases to sites supplied by the systemic circulation. Batson[2] postulated that cancer cells "short circuit" the capillaries of the lung through this system, which is formed by the mammary tributaries of the posterior intercostal veins flowing toward the vertebral plexus. They then pass along an efferent system of veins which drains from the vertebral plexus toward the sites of lodgment of the cancer cells in the head and the extremities.

LYMPHATIC DRAINAGE OF THE BREAST

The importance of lymphatic drainage of the breast lies in the spread of carcinoma. The anatomy of the aggregations of lymph nodes is important both for the surgical and radiotherapeutic management of the patient with a breast malignancy.

The lymphatic drainage of the breast is similar to that of other parts of the body. Lymph vessels accompany the blood supply. The largest amount of lymph drains along the lateral mammary vessels to the axillary and supraclavicular lymphatic chains.

The Main Lymphatic Pathway

Lymphatics arise adjacent to lobules of the breast and drain through the deep substance of the breast toward the axilla (Fig. 1-13). They extend along the axillary tail of the breast into the axilla, where they are joined by tributaries from the arm.

The main breast lymphatics run parallel to the lateral mammary vessels (lateral thoracic vessels) and drain into the anterior group of axillary nodes. A few lymphatics pass to the posterior group along the subscapular vein. From there lymph drains to central and apical groups which are situated around the inferomedial and anterior aspects of the axillary vein.[33] Hultborn[13] showed with the use of radioactive colloidal gold (^{198}Au) that in all cases, regardless of the site of the injection in the breast, some of the axillary lymph nodes showed an uptake of radiogold. This included all four quadrants, the central and subareolar parts of the breast, as well as the most medial parts of the breast.

Anastomosis of
superficial and
deep venous
systems

Superficial vein

Polygonal peri-
areolar vein

Bristles in
lactiferous ducts
of the nipple

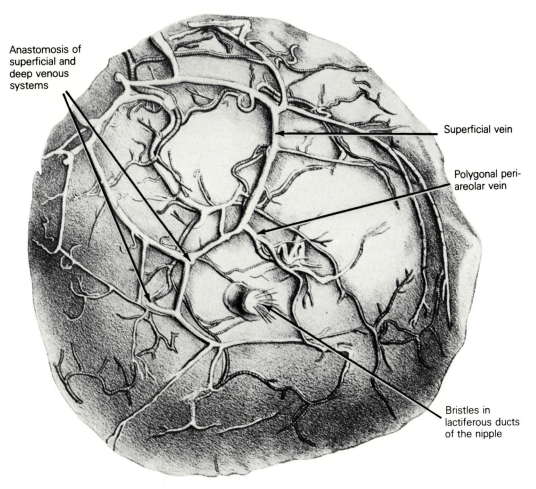

FIG. 1–12.

The superficial venous drainage of the breast. Sir Astley Cooper's illustration of a lactating breast with bristles placed in the lactiferous ducts of the nipple. The superficial veins are light colored. The periareolar venous anastomosis is polygonal in shape. (Cooper, A.: The Anatomy and Diseases of the Breast. Philadelphia, Lea & Blanchard, 1845)

Table 1-1. Percentages of Drainage in Breast Lymphatics From Several Mammary Areas

Site of [198]Au Injection	Axillary Nodes (%)	Internal Mammary Nodes (%)	Supraclavicular Nodes	Other
Upper inner quadrant	94	62	6	8
Lower inner quadrant	68	86	2	6
Upper outer quadrant	98	36	4	0
Lower outer quandrant	90	64	4	12
Subareolar region	100	20	0	2

(Vendrell-Torné, J., Setoain-Quinquer, J., and Doménech-Torné, F. M.: Study of normal mammary lymphatic drainage using radioactive isotopes. J. Nucl. Med., **13**: 801, 1972)

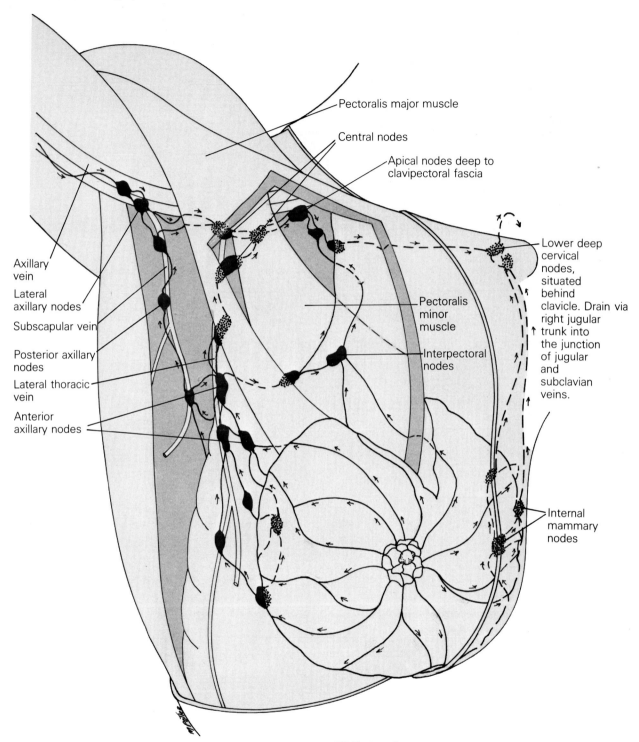

Pectoralis major muscle

Central nodes

Apical nodes deep to
clavipectoral fascia

Lower deep
cervical
nodes,
situated
behind
clavicle. Drain via
right jugular
trunk into
the junction
of jugular
and
subclavian
veins.

Axillary
vein

Lateral
axillary nodes

Subscapular vein

Posterior axillary
nodes

Lateral thoracic
vein

Anterior
axillary nodes

Pectoralis
minor
muscle

Interpectoral
nodes

Internal
mammary
nodes

FIG. 1–13.
The main lymphatic pathways. Most of the drainage is
along the axillary tail of the breast to the anterior group
and then to the apical group of lymph nodes.

Internal Mammary Lymph Nodes

Handley and Thackray[10] have described the anatomy of the internal mammary lymphatic chain. The internal mammary lymph nodes mostly receive lymph from the medial side of the breast, but also from all regions of the breast. Afferent lymphatics from the breast reach the chain by perforating the intercostal muscles, usually with the anterior perforating arteries of the internal mammary artery. The nodes lie posterior to the intercostal muscles and are inconstant both in position and in number. The chain begins in the sixth intercostal space where it drains the region of the diaphragm and the liver and ends behind the sternal head of the sternomastoid muscle, draining into a lymph node which discharges into the great veins. Nodes most frequently occur in the second space, followed in frequency by the first and third spaces. These vessels also receive lymph from vessels accompanying the lateral perforating branches of the upper intercostal vessels. Smaller posterior intercostal nodes are also found in the upper three or four intercostal spaces. These posterior lymph nodes lie behind the necks of the ribs, close to the vertebra.[33] These perforating lymphatics constitute a theoretical lymphatic communication between the axillary and internal mammary lymphatic pathways.

The perforating lymph vessels leave the posterior surface of the breast and pass through the pectoralis major to vessels lying between the pectoralis major and minor muscles. They then drain to the axillary or internal mammary nodes. No lymphatics penetrate the pectoralis minor muscle.

The Deep Fascial Plexus

There is no evidence to support the formerly held theory that mammary lymphatics communicate with the fine plexus which is found in the fascial plane. However, a few lymphatics do traverse the retromammary space, entering the pectoralis major muscle or the intercostal space.

The Subcutaneous Lymphatics

There is a subcutaneous lymphatic plexus which does not differ from other parts of the body. It lies in the same plane as the superficial venous plexus of the breast and extends and communicates with the skin surrounding the breast. There is reason to believe that carcinoma can spread in this plane, and therefore a wide margin of skin should be taken during the resection of a breast carcinoma.

The Subareolar Plexus of Sappey

In 1885, Sappey described this plexus which he thought drained the lobular system of the breast. The subcutaneous network in this area communicates with the lymphatics around the lactiferous ducts, but it does not represent an essential confluent point in the pathway of the lymphatic drainage of the breast.[33]

Contralateral Drainage

Under normal conditions, there is no significant drainage of lymph to the contralateral axilla or internal mammary chains.[33] Vendrell-Torné[34] found only two cases in 250 indirect mammary lymphoscintiscans which crossed the body midline. In these two cases, the flow was to the internal mammary nodes.

Gerota's Node

Vendrell-Torné[34] demonstrated flow to a Gerota's paramammarian node in seven out of 250 cases. The node is located in a vertical line dropped between the middle one-third and outer two-thirds of the clavicle. It belongs to the internal mammary lymphatic trunk and Vendrell-Torné demonstrated the sequence of radioactive nodes to the internal mammary nodes. In 1896, Gerota postulated lymphatic pathways which ran from the breast via intercostal spaces to the parasternal vessels.

The Distribution of Lymph Flow

The axillary lymph nodes are the main drainage center of mammary lymph, except for the lower inner quadrant where the lymph has a greater tendency to flow into the internal mammary nodes.[34] However, the internal mammary nodes are of greater importance than is generally considered. Most of the lymphatic drainage from the medial part of the breast drains to the internal mammary group, but it also drains all quadrants of the breast, including the subareolar area.

Hultborn and associates,[13] using radiogold (^{198}Au) and a scintillation counter, found that 85 per cent of the colloid remained at the site of the injection into the breast. In the cases where both

Augmentation mammaplasty is the most commonly performed breast operation, with several thousand of these procedures being performed each year in a rapidly increasing number of countries. This large number of operations is due, in part, to the natural desire of the underdeveloped female to have normal-sized breasts. Where full breasts have been for centuries a symbol of erotic femininity, there is also, on the part of many females, an urge to enlarge breasts of "normal" size. Occasionally, an inverted nipple further detracts from the appearance of the breasts, a condition which can be surgically improved.

The operation is conceptually simple and consists in almost all cases of insertion of an alloplastic implant between the pectoral muscle and the undersurface of the existing breast tissue (Fig. 2-1). This provides a greater bulk, and ideally a pleasing contour, to the breasts. The breasts should not only appear visually normal but, importantly, should also feel normal to palpation without the sensation of foreign objects beneath the hand.

HISTORIC ASPECTS

Augmentation mammaplasty, although simple, is a comparatively recent operative procedure.

The earliest operations involved the insertion or injection of various foreign substances, including liquid paraffin, oil, rubber, and other synthetics. Disillusionment with these crude procedures was rapid along with the obvious and, in some cases, severe complications such as skin necrosis and firm mass formation.

The pendulum swung away from alloplastic materials and toward the use of autogenous tissue only.

Longacre[8] described the use of dermal-fat flaps, taken from the inframammary region, and swung to repose behind the breast. This procedure, while yielding a fairly uniformly pleasing result, was limited in its scope of augmentation to produce a rather minimal increase in size (Figs. 2-2, 2-3).

The other principal use of autogenous tissue in augmentation mammaplasty has been the transplantation of a free graft, initially of fat and later of dermal-fat composite grafts.[14] This procedure involves a bilateral elliptical excision of portions of the buttocks or abdomen (Fig. 2-4). After de-epithelialization, the free graft is folded, dermal side outward, and inserted into a retromammary pocket. When successful, the results of this procedure are as pleasing as those of any procedure performed today (Fig. 2-5A, B). The principal drawbacks are (1) an unpredictable resorption of the graft, resulting, in many cases, in gross asymmetry, and (2) severe scarring of the donor region.

As the technology of the plastics industry led to improved materials, the pendulum swung back to the use of alloplastic materials in augmentation mammaplasty. Polyethylene balls[9] and sponges of Etheron,[11] Ivalon,[6] and Teflon[4] were used in large numbers during the 1950s. However, these also became hardened and deformed.

In the 1960s, two major advances in the art of breast augmentation were reported. One of these has stood the test of time, the other has not.

When physiologically inert silicone derivatives were introduced by the Dow-Corning Company, they were used in two ways.

Conway and his associates developed the method of direct injection of dimethylpolysiloxane liquid into the breast.[1] This procedure gave the most aesthetically pleasing results to date, making possible an augmentation of almost unlimited size with no sensation of "foreign body" beneath the tissues.

However, with the passage of time, many serious long-range complications have developed. These have varied from nodular compaction of the liquid within the breast to ischemia and frank gangrene of the skin resulting in some cases in the loss of the

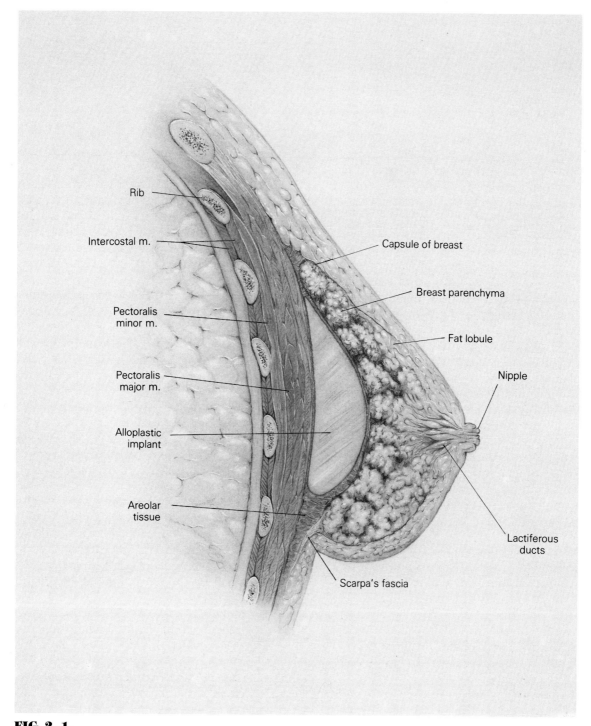

Rib

Intercostal m.

Capsule of breast

Breast parenchyma

Pectoralis
minor m.

Fat lobule

Pectoralis
major m.

Nipple

Alloplastic
implant

Areolar
tissue

Lactiferous
ducts

Scarpa's fascia

FIG. 2–1.
A lateral diagram of the augmented breast, showing the implant lying between the
pectoral muscle and the breast tissue.

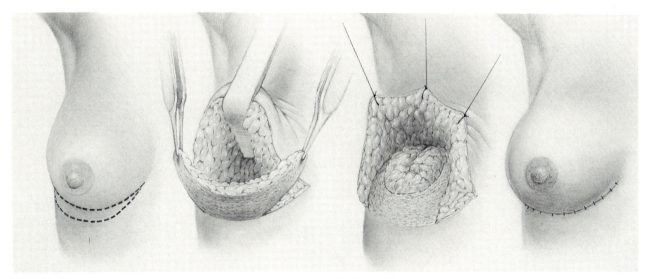

FIG. 2-2.
Longacre's technique for augmentation, using dermal-fat flaps from the inframammary region.

FIG. 2-3.
The flaps are mobilized and plicated behind the elevated breast tissue.

FIG. 2-4.
Free composite grafts are cut from the buttocks, de-ephithelialized, folded with the dermis side out, and placed in retromammary pocket.

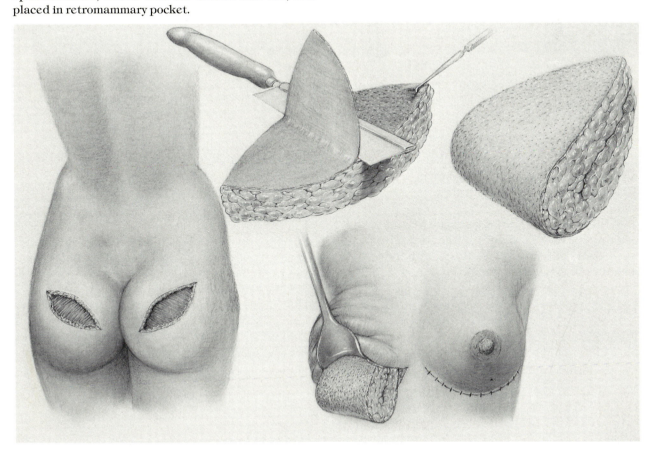

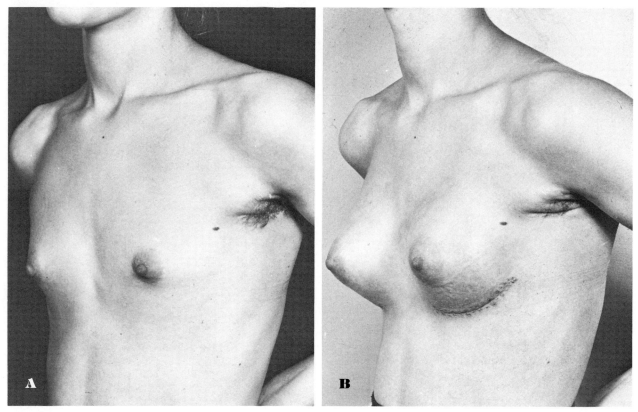

FIG. 2–5.
A. Preoperative view of a patient with micromastia. B. Following augmentation with bilateral free autogenous dermal-fat grafts.

entire breast (Fig. 2-6A, B, C). Faced with these devastating complications, the FDA in the mid-1960s declared the procedure unacceptable and illegal.

At the same time, Cronin and Gerow were investigating the use of a silastic gel contained in a preformed silastic capsule.[2] This implant, the Cronin prosthesis, is widely in use today.

CONTEMPORARY PROCEDURES

With few exceptions, the vast majority of breast augmentations performed today use variations of the preformed silastic gel implants described by Cronin. These variations include (1) the route of insertion of the implant and (2) different types of implant.

ROUTE OF INSERTION OF THE IMPLANT

The most commonly used incision for augmentation mammaplasty is the inframammary incision. Other recommended routes for insertion of the implant include an areolar approach, the axillary incision, and even an abdominal route where a lipectomy is performed (Fig. 2-7). Each method has advantages and drawbacks when compared with the more commonly used inframammary incision.

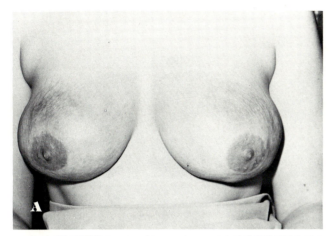

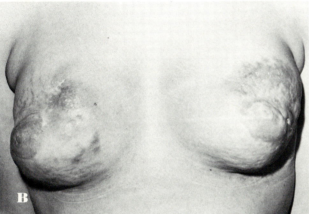

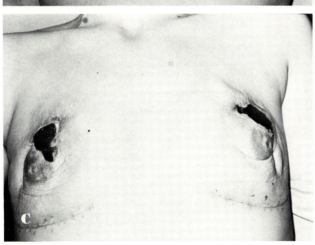

FIG. 2–6.
A. Erythema and dermal fibrosis four years after silicone injection. B. Progression, in the space of two years, to nodular deformity of the breasts and impending skin necrosis. C. Frank gangrene which has required subcutaneous mastectomy.

FIG. 2–7.
The most frequently used incisions for augmentation mammaplasty.

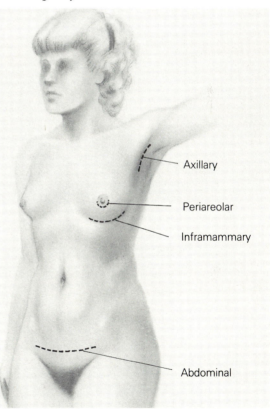

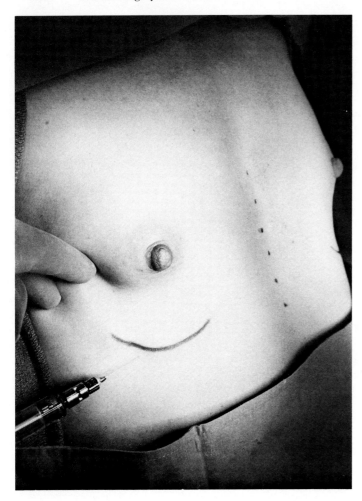

I-1
I-2

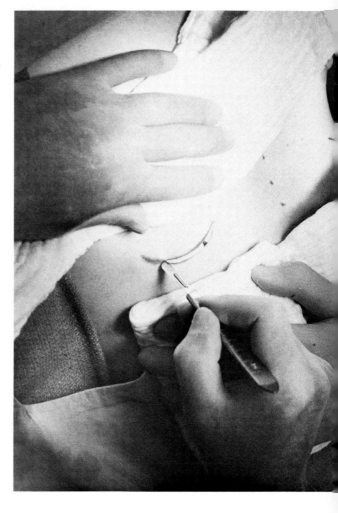

Inframammary Approach

In this procedure, a slightly curved incision is made directly below the nipple in the future inframammary fold (I-1, I-2). The incision is carried through to the pectoral fascia, and skin and subcutaneous hemostasis is achieved. The upper skin edge is then lifted up and with sharp dissection the inferior surface of the breast is lifted and separated from the pectoral fascia (I-3).

Having reached the level of the nipple, dissection can proceed bluntly. Ample pockets, larger than the implants, are developed to the midline, close to the clavicle, and beyond the lateral border of the breast (I-4). Significant bleeding may be encountered medially from perforators of the internal mammary vessels, laterally from branches of the lateral thoracic artery, and, hardest of all to stop due to their distance from the incision, vessels in the superior margin of the dissection.

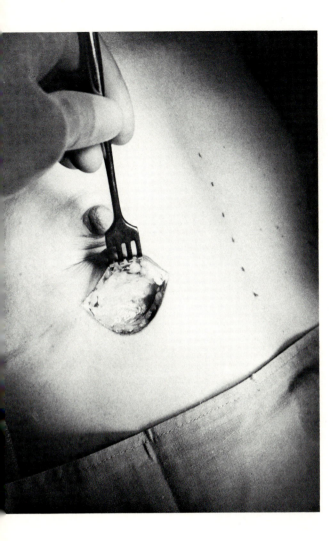

I-3
I-4

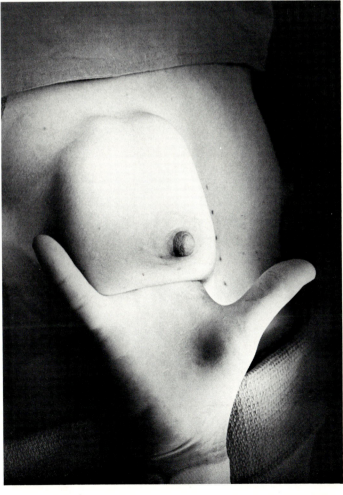

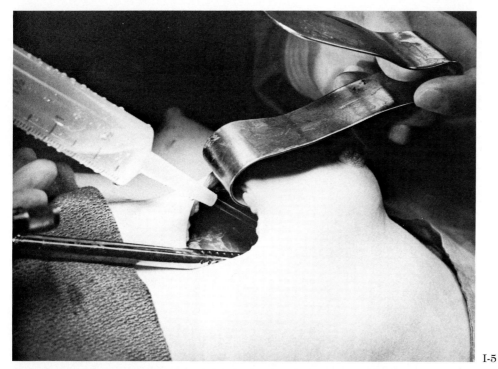

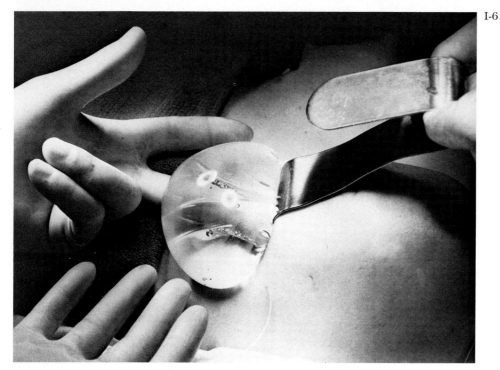

Having achieved hemostasis, the cavities are irrigated (I-5) and the prosthesis is inserted (I-6).

The incision is then closed in several layers (I-7), preferably using a subcuticular closure for the skin supported with Steri-Strips (I-8). Drainage (by a Penrose drain or Hemovac) is instituted only on those rare occasions where uncontrollable oozing is encountered; however, in the majority of cases no drainage is necessary.

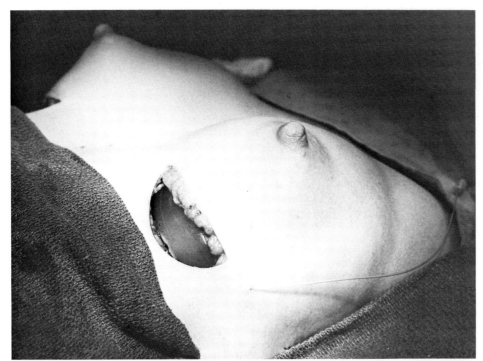

I-7

I-8

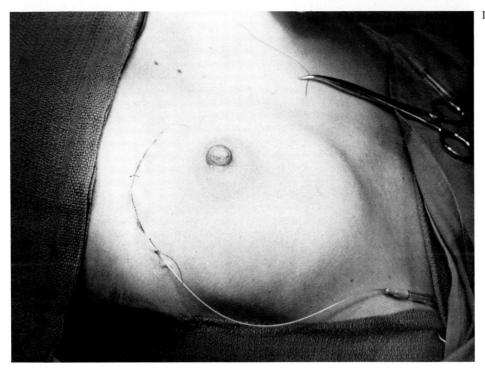

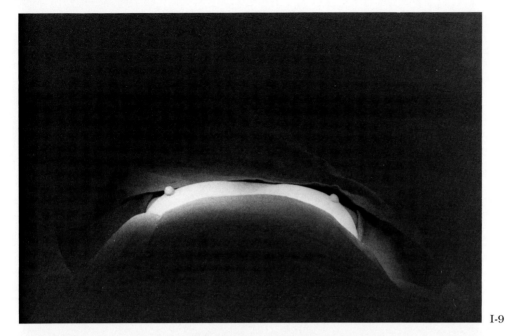

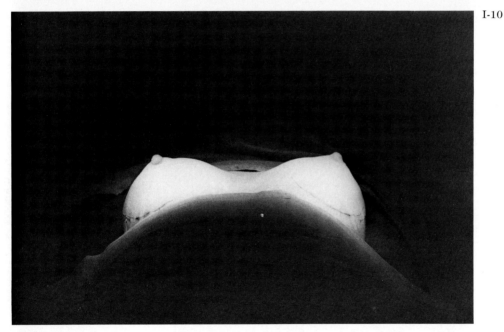

The breasts are then supported by a pressure dressing constructed either of Elasto-plast, Ace bandages, or a custom-designed elastic brassiere such as the Jobst Breast Support.

Pre- and postoperative views of the patient in the supine position are shown (I-9, I-10).

The skin sutures are removed a week postoperatively, and limitation of activity, particularly arm movement, is required for a month to permit rapid and unin-flamed healing around the implant.

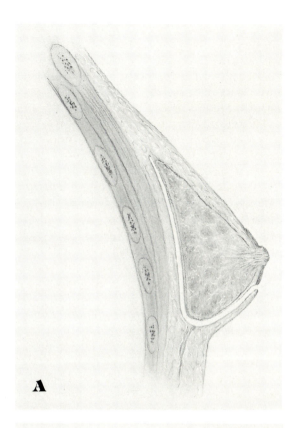

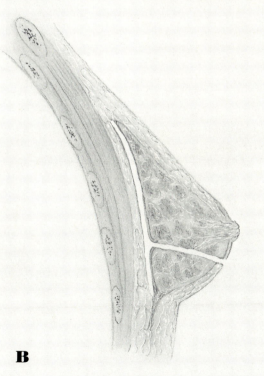

Areolar Approach

The areolar approach involves an incision around half the circumference of the nipple, usually the inferior half. Dissection may proceed inferiorly around the glandular portion of the breast until its inferior margin is reached, at which point the breast is separated from the pectoral fascia as before (Fig. 2-8A).

Alternatively, the breast tissue deep to the areolar incision may be incised until the plane of dissection between the breasts and pectoral fascia is reached. Blunt dissection then proceeds both superiorly and inferiorly until an adequate pocket is achieved (Fig. 2-8B). This incision carries with it the advantage of leaving almost no visible scar on the skin of the torso (Fig. 2-9).

FIG. 2–8.
A. Periareolar incision with the plane of dissection around the inferior pole of the breast. B. Periareolar incision with dissection through the breast to gain access to the retromammary pocket.

FIG. 2–9.
The scar resulting from the periareolar approach is usually inconspicuous.

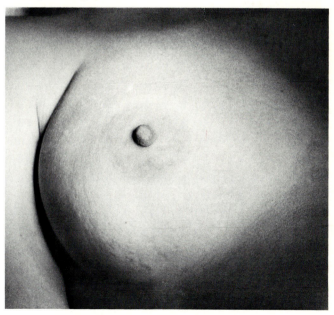

The main disadvantage arises from the fact that, when the breast tissue itself is incised, scarring occurs in the substance of the breast which in later years is hard to distinguish from breast masses. Where the areolar incision is followed by a dissection around the bulk of the glandular portion of the breast, bruising of the skin is quite marked and the exposure is limited, making identification and ligation of bleeding points at the upper pole of the breast cavity difficult.

Axillary and Abdominal Approaches

The axillary approach, while affording an equally inconspicuous skin incision, suffers from the same drawbacks as the areolar approach, namely that exposure is limited and hemostasis is very difficult if there are distant awkward bleeders.

The abdominal approach has the same limitations and is employed even more rarely.

TYPE OF IMPLANT

The main types of prostheses are the silastic gel-filled implant, the inflatable implant, and the double-lumen implant (Fig. 2-10).

Gel-Filled Implants

These implants are all derived from the original Cronin implant and may be ordered with or without a fabric fixation patch. Different manufacturers claim advantages for their own particular modifications aimed at achieving a contour and "feel" as close to natural as possible. Ultimately the type of implant used depends on the personal preference of the surgeon.

Because all the gel-filled implants are of a predetermined size, numerous models are employed. These vary in size from 75 cc. to 450 cc. in order to accommodate individuals of different body habitus and varying objectives in terms of enlargement. The surgeon must beware of undertaking too ambitious a procedure; an overly large implant will yield a tight pocket and an unnatural-appearing breast, with varying degrees of discomfort to the patient.

The majority of implants used are in the range of from 200 cc. to 300 cc.

The two basic shapes of implants employed are the tear drop and the round, or hemispheric, prosthesis; an intermediary shape, low-profile, is available from some manufacturers (Fig. 2-11A, B, C).

The tear drop prosthesis, shaped somewhat like a pendulous normal breast, is used principally to augment breasts of persons with marked hypomastia and almost no feminine contour to the torso (Fig. 2-12A, B).

The round, or hemispheric, prosthesis is used to augment breasts of individuals with a shape characteristic of postpartum breast atrophy. The

FIG. 2–10.
An inflatable implant and a gel-filled prosthesis of equivalent size.

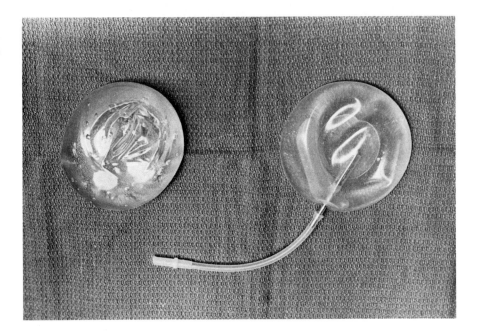

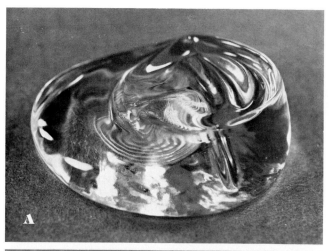

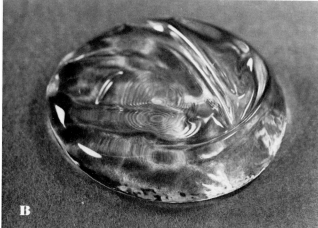

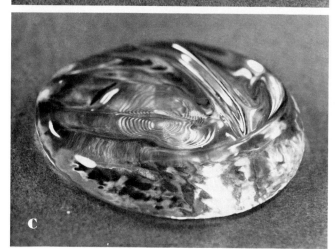

FIG. 2–11.
A. The tear drop, or contour, prosthesis. B. The round (more accurately, hemispheric) prosthesis. C. The low-profile prosthesis, intermediate between A and B.

rounder implant fills in the upper aspect of the breast, giving a convex contour and cleavage to the breasts which have sustained atrophy and moderate ptosis (Fig. 2-13A, B).

Intermediate between these two is the low-profile design (Fig. 2-14A, B).

Inflatable Implants

The other principal method of augmentation mammaplasty employs an empty silastic sack which may be filled with saline through a valve.[13] Inflation is carried out until the desired size is reached. Obviously, no predetermined shape can be achieved with this type of implant.

The advantages of inflatable implants include the need for a much smaller incision (either periareolar or a 1-inch inframammary incision). Augmentation to the exact size desired is possible without resorting to the compromise inherent in a fixed-size prosthesis. This is particularly useful in cases of mild asymmetry.

The disadvantages include occasional leakage through the valve with subsequent loss of the bulk achieved.[5] In thin people with a meager amount of breast tissue, the valve may be palpable through the prosthesis. The sack itself is slightly firmer than the more recent "thin-walled" gel-filled models and thus is more readily discernible as a foreign object.

Double-Lumen Implants

These implants are a relatively recent modification, not in widespread use now, and consist of an inner sack of fixed size filled with silastic gel, to which is added an outer lumen which is inflatable with saline through a valve.[7] The outer lumen is inflated to the desired volume upon introduction of the prosthesis, and, if no untoward reactions occur, is left as is. If, however, a scar contracture develops (see Complications, below), the surgeon

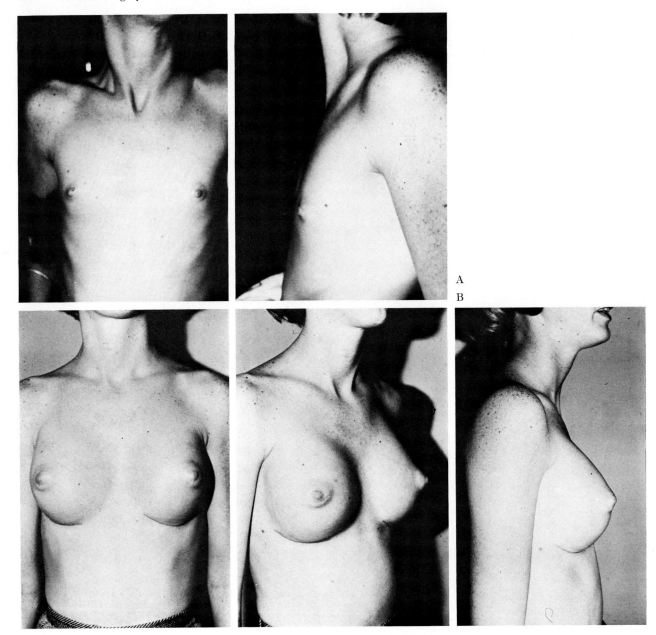

FIG. 2–12.
A. A young female with almost complete breast agenesis and a totally unfeminine chest contour. B. Following augmentation with contoured prosthesis, which yielded a natural and pleasing appearance.

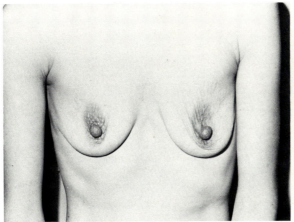
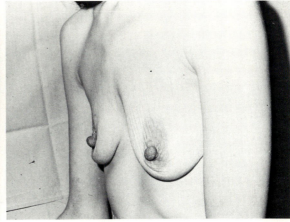

A

B

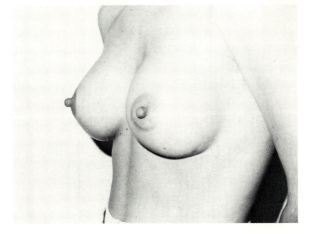

FIG. 2–13.
A. Marked postpartum atrophy with borderline ptosis.
B. Restitution of volume and contour with hemispheric prosthesis.

can make a small incision and withdraw saline from the outer lumen, resulting in a smaller implant than was originally planned for. The implant will be under less tension and consequently will be less firm. Although this method seems a logical answer to the problem of scar contracture, there has not yet been enough follow-up to judge its ultimate value.

An additional modification to this concept has been developed by Perrin, and consists of filling the outer lumen with dilute steroid solution.[10] The outer capsule acts as a semipermeable membrane, allowing the steroid to diffuse into the tissues surrounding the implant. This long-range steroid release will theoretically hinder the tendency of the body to form scar tissue around the implant, by virtue of the known effects of local steroids upon collagen synthesis.

COMPLICATIONS

Although the procedure of augmentation mammaplasty is, as can be seen from the preceding descriptions, a basically simple technical exercise, subtle pitfalls lurk in wait for the unwary, casual, or inexperienced surgeon. These complications may produce a result that is totally unsatisfactory, leading to great unhappiness on the part of both patient and surgeon. Such complications may be arbitrarily classified as immediate, early, and late.

IMMEDIATE COMPLICATIONS

These complications result from lack of judgment on the part of the operating surgeon and are apparent as soon as the operation is completed. The result is predestined to be unacceptable.

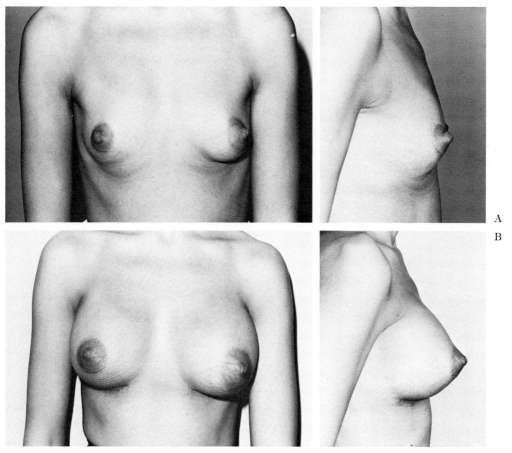

A
B

FIG. 2–14.
A. Moderate postpartum atrophy superimposed upon already quite small breasts—
the commonest clinical situation. B. Satisfactory contour achieved with low-profile
prosthesis.

Oversized Implant

The most common immediate complication is the
selection of too large an implant. This will be mani-
fested by tightness of the skin and varying degrees
of long-range discomfort to the patient. Also,
the contour of the breast will be inappropriate.

The implants, either gel-filled or saline-inflat-
able, increase in all three dimensions as their size
progresses. Too large an implant may be too "tall"
for a person of short stature, resulting in a breast
contour that juts out directly below the clavicle.
The implant may be too wide for slender women
and project laterally under their axillae due to the
angulation of the narrower rib cage.

Most patients seeking augmentation mammaplasty ask for one of two general degrees of augmentation. Either they express the wish to have a
modest increment which yields them a feminine
contour without being obviously a great deal
larger, or, an equally valid desire, they want to
have an augmentation that is as large as can be accomplished with safety. In the first instance, the
patient's desire can easily be satisfied without jeo-
pardizing the success of the operation. In the second situation, the surgeon must be the limiting factor as to what degree the patient's breasts can be
augmented. The surgeon himself, rather than the
patient, must determine the size of the implant to
be used to achieve the maximum degree of aug-

mentation possible without running into the complications listed above.

In general, we use the rough rule of thumb that females of small and slender stature may be augmented with an implant of up to 200 cc. with security. A person of medium build (up to 5 ft. 6 in. and 120 lb.) may be augmented up to 300 cc.; persons of large stature who desire maximum augmentation may take implants from 300 cc. to 400 cc. In our series, very rarely have prostheses of over 400 cc. been implanted.

Inadequate Dissection

A second immediate complication, related indirectly to the above, is the inadequate dissection of pockets large enough for the size of the implants chosen. This mistake, common among neophytes in the field, leads to the same degree of discomfort and tight, hard-feeling implants which are under excessive pressure from the surrounding soft tissue and skin.

Improper Placement

Very rarely, the implants may be placed improperly, resulting in an inappropriate or even asymmetric feminine contour. Most prostheses come with detailed instructions on the placing of the implants. These instructions should be followed exactly for the best results. When inframammary incisions are placed too low, they end up in a very egregious position on the chest wall, visible below the underseam of the upper half of a two-piece bathing suit or a brassiere.

EARLY COMPLICATIONS

These complications occur in the first three days following surgery, and the most common, hemorrhage, is almost always manifest in the first 24 hours. Infection, a rare but disastrous complication, will also usually show its earliest signs and symptoms (pain, fever, redness of the suture line) during this period.

Hemorrhage and Hematoma

The principal early complication is postoperative hemorrhage or hematoma resulting from an unnoticed intraoperative bleeding point. Early postoperative hemorrhage is usually evident within several hours of surgery. The outward manifestation

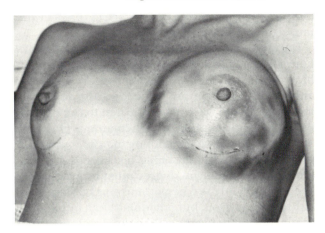

FIG. 2–15.
Swelling and ecchymosis characteristic of an acute hematoma.

of this complication is, of course, swelling and discoloration of the skin overlying the dissection (Fig. 2-15). For this reason, the dressings **must** be checked on the evening of surgery. I prefer, therefore, to have the patient in the hospital overnight following the operation.

In order to minimize the likelihood of postoperative hemorrhage, we utilize the following procedure for hemostasis. After dissecting the first retromammary pocket, pack it with one or two "lap pads." Then dissect the pocket on the other side and pack it similarly. Remove the lap pads and copiously irrigate with normal saline to flush any small blood clots remaining from the dissection. Perform a complete inspection of the cavity with a fiberoptic retractor; any oozing vessels must be clamped, cauterized, and suture-ligated if necessary.

Institute Hemovac drainage if there is an uncontrollable slow ooze from the muscle. Check the volume of drainage every two hours by emptying the collapsible canister of the vacuum drain device. **The operation is never completed until hemostasis is secured.**

There were nine cases of postoperative hematoma in our series of 850 operations—a 1 per cent incidence, small but significant. In each case, the patient was returned to the operating room, the incisions were opened, the prosthesis was removed, and the cavity irrigated and inspected. In only four cases was there a discrete bleeding point which could be identified. The majority of cases showed

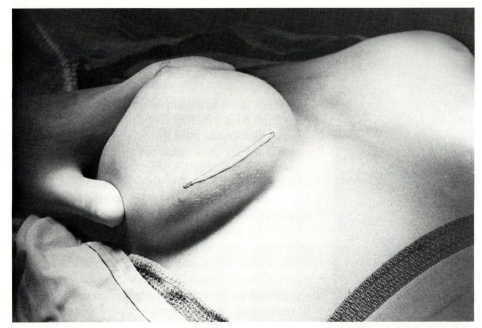

II-1

II-2

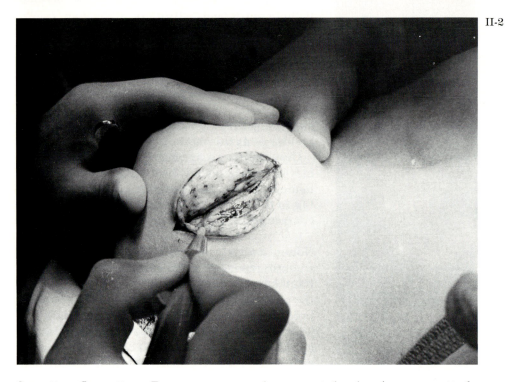

Operative Correction. Denser scar capsules cannot be lysed nonoperatively and therefore require surgical correction. The incision (II-1), either submammary or periareolar, is reopened and the capsule identified. It may be incised using the cutting current of an electrocoagulation unit (II-2), because this current will not damage the implant but will neatly sever the overlying capsule (II-3), allowing the implant to be removed (II-4).

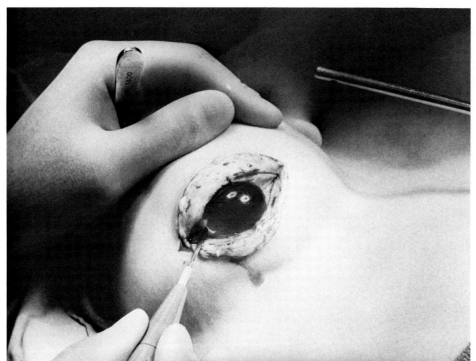

II-3

II-4

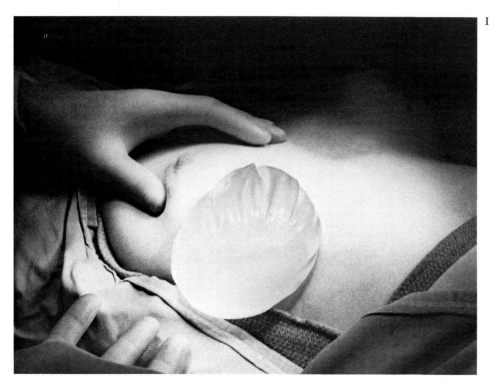

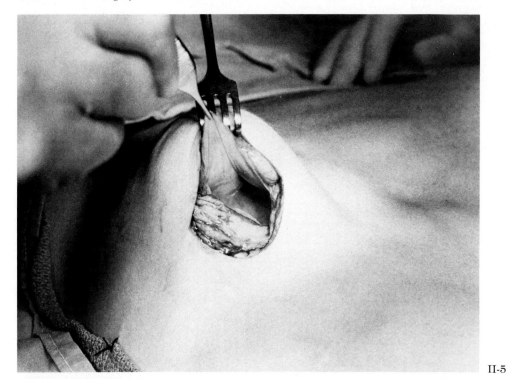

II-5

II-6

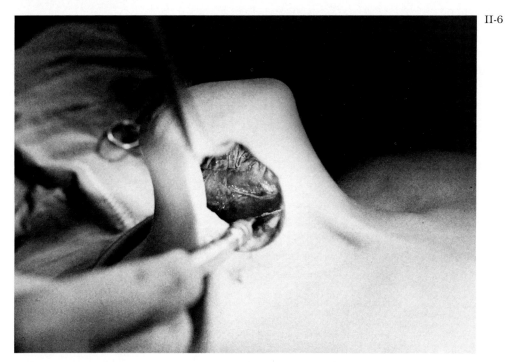

Having gained access to the entire scar capsule (II-5), its "cap" is either re-moved or crosshatched, allowing it to spread (II-6). Soft tissue dissection is carried out around the periphery of the pocket (II-7) to allow an overly large, loose, soft tissue enclosure for the implant.

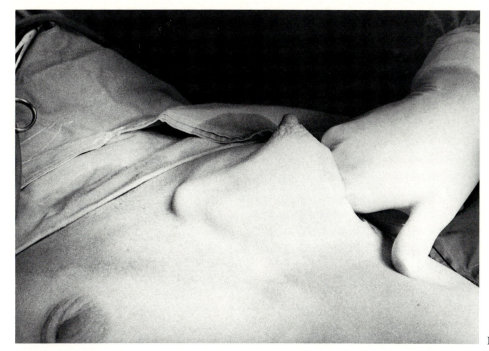

II-7

II-8

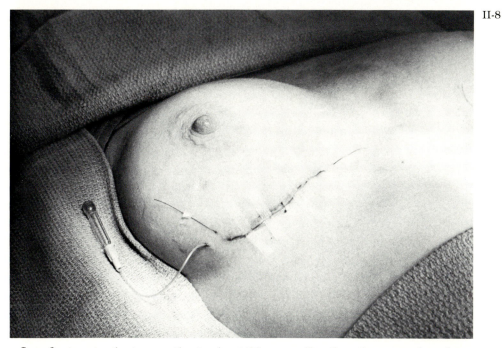

I prefer to reimplant a prosthesis about 50 cc. smaller than the original implant, allowing for a possible subsequent contracture with less firmness resulting. Instillation of a steroid is accomplished by means of leaving an Intra-Cath within the cavity (II-8) and instilling 125 mg. of Aristocort per side 24 hours following surgery. Although this maneuver has not been justified experimentally, it is felt to be useful in the prevention of a subsequent contracture.[15] This procedure almost always results in complete alleviation of the problem, although very rarely a second contracture may develop.

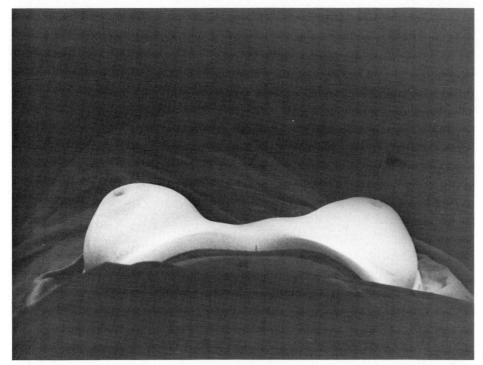

II-9

II-10

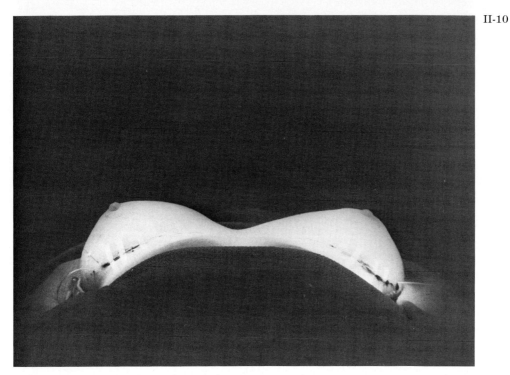

Pre- and postoperative views of the patient in the supine position are shown (II-9, II-10).

In summary, this, the most common complication of augmentation mammaplasty, is still a mysterious and unpredictable phenomenon. Although factors such as excessive motion with shearing of tissue planes, hematoma, and subclinical infection have all been implicated by various authors, the cause-and-effect relationship between these factors and the development of a scar capsule has not been demonstrated either in the laboratory or clinically. In addition, the possibility of imperfect quality control in the manufacturing process of the implants, producing contaminants leading to an intense foreign-body reaction, has to be considered, together with an ill-defined "spectrum of patient reactivity."

AUTHOR'S CHOICE OF PROCEDURE

At the time of writing, approximately 850 augmentation mammaplasties for symmetrical micromastia or postpartum breast atrophy have been performed by the author, the majority in the past four years. Certain inescapable conclusions have been reached as a result of a review of this series, and these will be discussed in terms of the principal controversies surrounding the procedure.

INFRAMAMMARY APPROACH

In general, the inframammary approach is considered superior to the two other principal routes of insertion and has been employed in the majority of our cases. The principal considerations involving this decision have been the following:

The exposure to the submammary pocket is far easier in the inframammary approach than in either the areolar or axillary approach. The entire pocket can be visualized and hemorrhage at the furthest reaches of the dissection can be readily controlled.

With no surgical interference of the glandular portion of the breast, there is no scarring in the breast itself and no interruption of the ductal system leading to the nipple. This obviates scarring within the breast which may be mistaken for a subsequent breast mass; nursing of a baby, although not recommended, is entirely possible and has been successfully carried out by several of our patients following breast augmentation.

The incision, which is about two inches long and should be placed directly in (or just above) the in-

framammary crease, is, after scar maturation, very inconspicuous. Although the areolar incision is theoretically more aesthetically acceptable, in a few cases it has healed irregularly to yield a puckered scar requiring revision.

The resultant hidden nature of the axillary approach is not felt to be warranted in view of the relative length and "blindness" of the dissection. Significant bleeding may in fact be encountered in areas as far as ten inches from the incision.

GEL-FILLED IMPLANT

Both inflatable saline and fixed-mass gel-filled implants have been employed (Fig. 2-10). I prefer the gel-filled implants because the large variety of sizes and shapes available renders unimportant the advantage of being able to fill the implant to the exact degree required.

The saline implant represented a technical improvement over the older models of gel-filled implant which had a thick wall and a bonded seam which was, on occasion, palpable through the skin. However, the improved technology of manufacturing a seamless, thin-walled implant makes the gel-filled implant slightly less conspicuous than the firmer inflatable prosthesis. No leakages or rupture have been noted with the gel-filled prosthesis, whereas leakage was fairly common in the saline-filled implants.

FIXATION PATCHES

Patches of woven Dacron mesh may be bonded by the manufacturer to the flat underside of the gel-filled implant. I have used implants both with and without fixation patches.

Although the foreign body reaction excited by fixation patches has been blamed by many authors as a prime cause of scar contracture development, no difference whatsoever has been noted in our series between those procedures where fixation was employed and in those procedures where it was not. The principal advantage of fixation is that the implants adhere to the fascia of the pectoral muscle; thus, the weight of the implant is taken up entirely by its adhesion rather than being an extra strain on the skin envelope of the breast. The unfixed implants will theoretically allow an unsupported mass to exert a gravity effect on the skin of the breast. Although our studies have not been lengthy enough to demonstrate this phenomenon, it is felt to be an important consideration that, as the skin loses its tone and elasticity, this extra-weight would tend to produce ptosis of the augmented breast.

RECONSTRUCTION OF THE INVERTED NIPPLE

The inverted or retracted nipple may occur as a congenital defect, frequently associated with micromastia, or it may develop later in life as the skin of the breast becomes ptotic. In the latter situation, the surgeon should always suspect breast carcinoma, particularly where the retraction occurs unilaterally. Careful palpation for a mass directly beneath the nipple should be performed, and even if no mass is identified, a tissue specimen of breast in the immediate locality should be sent, at surgical correction, to the pathology laboratory for histologic examination.

Surgical correction of the inverted nipple has received surprisingly little attention in the breast literature, for the condition is both psychologically and funtionally disabling. Methods of correction have ranged from the ultra-simple—prolonged suction—to the complex. Skoog's[12] quite elaborate reconstruction is a good example of the latter, and is designed to permit the patient to nurse (often a compelling reason to seek correction); however, in our opinion this operation ignores the fact that the underlying pathology is shortening of the ducts leading from the glandular breast to the nipple eminence. Failure to divide these fore-shortened ducts will inevitably lead to a disappointing long-range result, with recurrence of the problem.

The procedure which we have found to be the most effective involves the sectioning of these ducts as an integral part of the operation. For this reason it should only be employed upon those patients who have no desire subsequently to nurse.

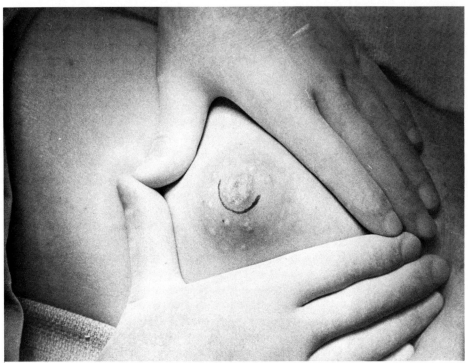

III-1

Under local or general anesthesia, a semicircular incision is made within the areola (III-1). This should be placed so that it will lie at the base of the cylindrical nipple and occupy one half of its circumference.

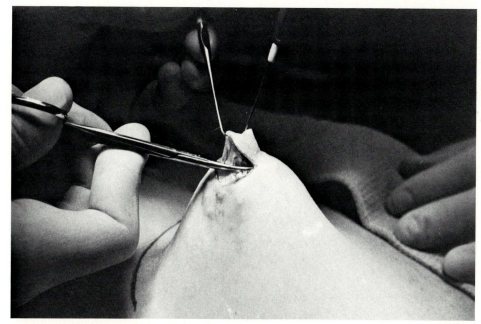

III-2

III-3

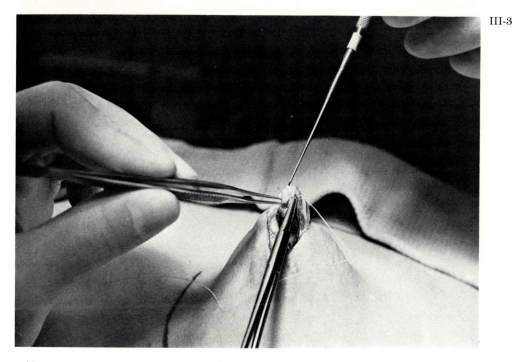

The sunken center of the nipple is identified and elevated with a skin hook above the surface of the adjacent areolar skin. The nipple is undermined, with sectioning of the ducts as necessary, until the nipple is completely freed with no tension pulling it back (III-2). The dermis of the nipple is then freed and plicated to itself in a vertical fashion (III-3) until a slight overcorrection of the nipple eminence has been achieved (III-4).

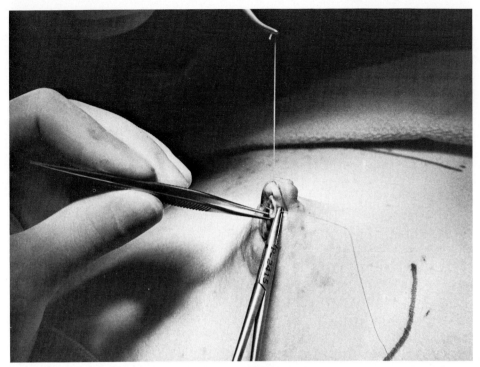

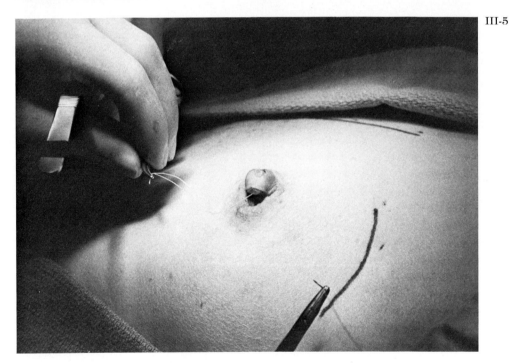

The nipple is allowed to fall back in place (III-5), and the semicircular incision is closed with a subcuticular nylon suture (III-6). The ends of this suture are then crossed behind the nipple and carefully pulled on to achieve a "purse-string" effect and further elevate the nipple (III-7). Great care must be taken not to strangle the nipple during this maneuver, and the dressing should be such that the color of the nipple can be watched postoperatively. Any hint of cyanosis or venous engorgement mandates the immediate loosening of the purse-string suture.

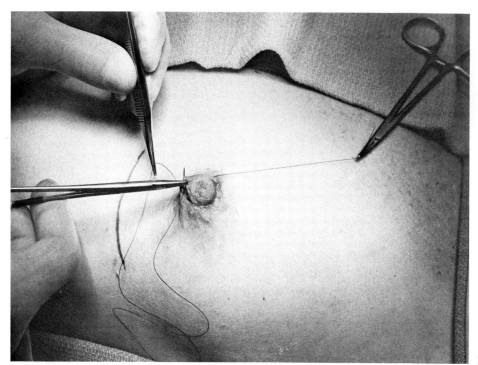

III-6

III-7

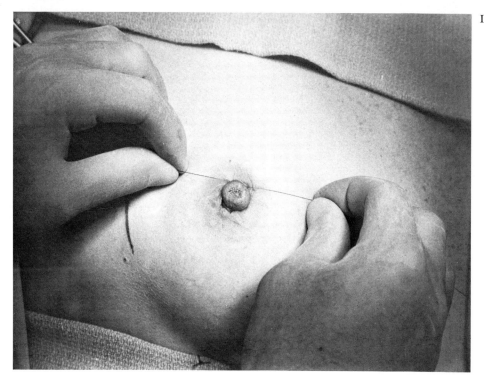

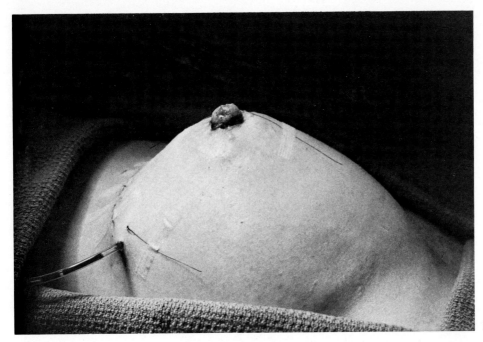

III-8

In III-8, an augmentation mammaplasty has been performed in conjunction with nipple reconstruction.

This simple procedure has been successful in our hands. There has not been a single long-range recurrence of the inversion in those patients with adequate follow-up. A representative case (with augmentation) is shown in Figure 2-18A and B.

HOSPITALIZATION

With increasing hospital costs, there is tremendous economic pressure to perform augmentation mammaplasty in as inexpensive a setting as possible. For this reason, many surgeons are performing the operation in either the outpatient department of the hospital or in an operating suite adjacent to their office.

I do not take any strong position in this regard, but prefer the security of having the patient in the hospital overnight. There, bed rest will make the development of early complications (particularly hemorrhage) less likely; proximity and easier monitoring of the patient in the hospital will allow these complications to be more easily recognized and dealt with. In our practice, the patient is admitted in the morning (having had the appropriate blood studies performed the day before), operated on under general anesthesia, and discharged (in most cases) the following morning. This limits the hospital stay to 24 hours—which, at the present time, is within the economic range of most patients. Occasionally patients will prefer to stay longer.

POSTOPERATIVE IMMOBILIZATION

Over the years I have become increasingly convinced that development of the scar tissue contracture is largely, although not exclusively, related to unwarranted movement of the arms in the first few weeks following surgery. With fixation patches, a foreign body reaction is provoked which forms fibrous adhesions between the mesh work of the patches and the pectoral fascia. If left undisturbed, this heals uneventfully; if unwarranted movement of the pectoral muscle causes shearing between the implant and the fascia, these tenuous connections will be disrupted and healing will be complicated by inflammation, serous accumulation, and quite rapid development of a scar tissue capsule.

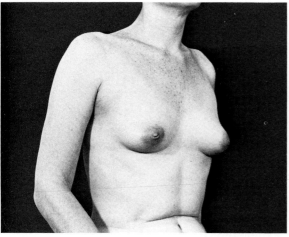
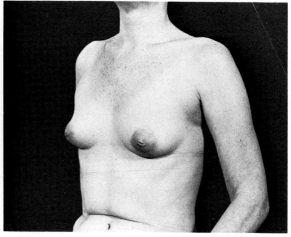

FIG. 2–18.
A. A preoperative case of inverted nipples with micromastia. B. Showing good nipple projection and insignificant scarring.

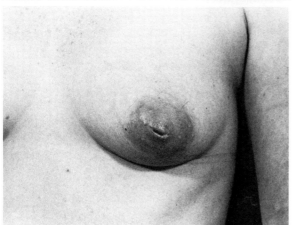

A
B

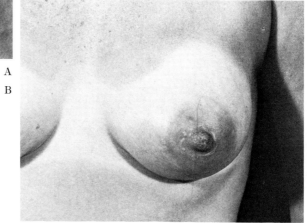

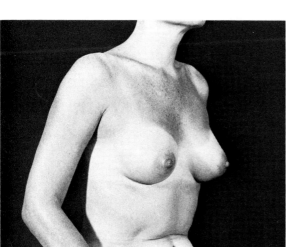
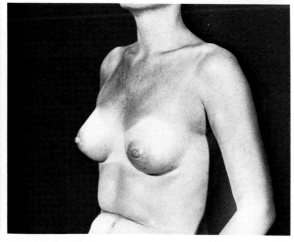

We now prescribe an extremely strict and inflexible program of limitation of activities to prevent this untoward occurrence:

1. **Days 1 through 10.** For the first 10 days, the patient is to be regarded as totally convalescent, pursuing a program of bed-sofa-chair, with activities limited to reading and watching television. If the patient has infants or young children (under the age of 3), it is insisted upon that she does not play any active part in the care and management of them for 10 days. If these conditions cannot be met, the operation is deferred.
2. **Days 11 through 20.** For the second 10 days of convalescence, light activity such as dusting and elementary cooking are permitted. Driving a car is not allowed for two weeks, and women who are in physically undemanding occupations can return to work at the end of this period.
3. **Days 21 through 35.** The fourth and fifth weeks of convalescence involve gradually resuming normal activity, with the exception of lifting, stretching, and any athletic endeavors.

At the end of six weeks the patient can resume a normal life with the exception of athletics involving marked arm activity such as tennis, bowling, volley ball, and cross-country skiing. These activities are deferred until such time as they excite no untoward reaction. Sexual activity involving the breasts should be avoided for the same period of time. With the rigid insistence upon this program of convalescence we have succeeded in cutting the incidence of postoperative scar tissue contracture from 12 per cent in the first four years of the series to 3½ per cent in the most recent four years. We feel so strongly about the efficacy of this program that unless the patient promises complete cooperation, we will not perform the operation.

Be it as it may, a small but significant incidence of scar capsular formation is, at this date, inevitable—and must be thoroughly explained to the patient contemplating augmentation mammaplasty.

REFERENCES

1. **Conway HC, Goulian D:** Experience with an injectable silastic R.T.V. as a subcutaneous material. Plast Reconstr Surg 32:294, 1963
2. **Cronin TD, Gerow FJ:** Augmentation mammaplasty: a new "natural-feel" prosthesis, Trans III. Int Congr Plast Surg 41:1964
3. **DeCholnoky T:** Augmentation mammaplasty: a survey of complications of 10,941 patients by 265 surgeons. Plast Reconstr Surg 45:573, 1970
4. **Edwards BF:** Teflon-silicone breast implants. Plast Reconstr Surg 32:519, 1963
5. **Grossman AR:** The current status of augmentation mammaplasty. Plast Reconstr Surg 52:1, 1973
6. **Harris HI:** Dermofat and Ivalon sponge for the correction of the hypoplastic breast Trans I. Int Congr Plast Surg 387:1957
7. **Hartley JH:** Specific applications of the double-lumen prosthesis. Clin Plast Surg 3:247, 1976
8. **Longacre JJ:** The use of local pedicle flaps for reconstruction of the breast. Plast Reconstr Surg 11:380, 1953
9. **Malbec EF:** Mammary hypoplasia, correction implants, Trans III. Int Congr Plast Surg 60:1964
10. **Perrin ER:** The use of soluble steroids within inflatable breast prostheses. Plast Reconstr Surg 57:163, 1976
11. **Regnault P:** One hundred cases of retromammary implantation of Etheron, Trans III. Congr Plast Surg 74:1964
12. **Skoog T:** Plastic Surgery. Stockholm, Almquist & Wiksell, 1974
13. **Tabari K:** Augmentation mammaplasty with simaplast implant. Plast Reconstr Surg 44:468, 1969
14. **Watson J:** Some observations of free fat grafts. Br J Plast Surg 12:263, 1960
15. **Williams JE:** Experiences with a large series of breast implants. Plast Reconstr Surg 49:253, 1972

3

reduction mammaplasty

Although there are technical similarities, reduction mammaplasty in this chapter is considered separately from mammapexy, or elevation of a purely ptotic breast, because reduction mammaplasty involves a diminution of bulk as well as correction of contour. It is the increased breast mass, rather than the accompanying skin laxity, which gives rise to the symptom complex for which correction is sought.

The condition for which this procedure is used goes by many different names. These include breast hypertrophy, macromastia, and even gigantomastia. All of these are, of course, anatomic descriptions rather than pathologic analyses of a true disease entity.

Breast hypertrophy, in addition to the severe psychological and social handicaps that it entails, such as the difficulty of purchasing properly fitting clothing and the embarrassment the affected individual feels in swimming attire or other sportswear, also has associated physical symptomatology. These include a stooped posture with frequent osteoarthritis of the cervical spine, intertrigo and other hygiene problems, and pressure grooves leading to dermatitis over the shoulders. For these reasons, correction of this deformity is eminently justified.

If descriptions of the clinical entity are numerous, operations described to correct it are overwhelming in number. At least one paper per year is published describing a new technique which, on close inspection, is merely a minor modification of an already established procedure. There are, however, certain papers which rank as "historical landmarks," such as those of Thorek,[10] Biesenberger,[1] Strombeck,[9] and Penn,[6] which will be referred to later. This state of confusion, implying that there is no one optimal procedure, has advantages as well as drawbacks. Whereas the neophyte is frustrated by the lack of a "party line," the experienced surgeon, wise in the handling of tissue and instinctive in his grasp of blood supply, may eclectically draw from all sources to evolve a comfortable procedure affording consistently good results.

There is much challenge and excitement in reduction mammaplasty, invoking the classic description of plastic surgery by Sir Harold Gillies, "a constant battle between beauty and blood supply." There is almost no other situation in plastic surgery where this apparently facetious comment is so apt, for unless judicious tension is preplanned into the operation—tension which, if exceeded, causes vascular compromise—the results will be flabbily mediocre. This challenge accounts for the indefatigable outpouring of intellectual energy by plastic surgeons the world over in an effort to achieve the perfect breast.

And yet, in my own personal experience, experience confirmed almost unanimously by other plastic surgeons, patients, from the adolescent with virginal breast hypertrophy to the middle-aged woman with massive pendulous breasts, are uniformly grateful for the ending of discomfort caused by excessive breast bulk. This gratitude in general overwhelms purely aesthetic considerations such as visible scarring, modest asymmetry, and loss of nipple sensation. These complications are generally more distressing to the surgeon than to the patient.

HISTORIC ASPECTS

Early techniques of reduction mammaplasty involved the resection of wedges of skin and breast tissue from above or below the nipple (Fig. 3-1), the latter being somewhat superior from the standpoint of visible scarring but both being crude and unacceptable compared with techniques in use today. The history of early attempts at reduction mammaplasty has been described most thoroughly by several authors; the reader's attention is directed to the review by Serafin in 1976.[8] A brief mention of the major historical landmarks is, however, in order.

In 1922, Thorek[10] advocated amputation of redundant breast tissue, sculpturing of the residual, and a free nipple transfer. This procedure with modifications is widely in use today.

In the same decade, Lexer,[4] Biesenberger,[1] and Joseph[3] all described procedures in which skin was resected and widely undermined to free it from the underlying breast; the nipple was transposed superiorly without being detached from its dermal base; the gland was reduced and shaped conically. A quite common complication of this procedure was slough of either the nipple or breast skin itself.

In 1960, Strombeck[9] opened up new vistas of security for plastic surgeons concerned with the high rate of complications with older nipple-transposing techniques. He devised a procedure using a Wise pattern for skin marking and preserving the nipple's vascular integrity on a horizontal dermal breast "bridge." This procedure led to modifications by McKissock,[5] Penn,[6,7] and others who have refined the technique to avoid both the squarish

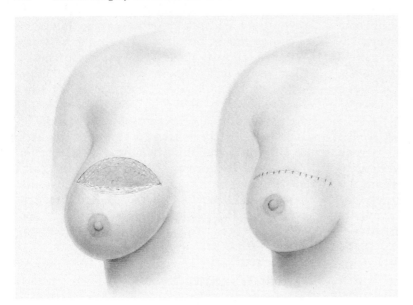

FIG. 3–1.
An historic and somewhat crude breast reduction.

contour and rather noticeable scarring which may result from the Strombeck procedure when applied in a "cut on the dotted line" fashion.

CONTEMPORARY PROCEDURES

Procedures in use today can be broadly divided into two groups: (1) those which employ a resection of breast and skin with a free nipple graft; and (2) various nipple-transposition techniques.

RESECTION OF BREAST AND SKIN WITH FREE NIPPLE GRAFT

This operation was first described in English in 1922 by Thorek,[10] and with minor modifications (principally those of Conway[2]) is used widely today.

Indications

The principal indication for use of this procedure is in cases where truly massive hypertrophy, or severe ptosis, is such that dermal flaps cut to support the nipple would be too bulky to fit into the residual skin envelope after appropriate resection. Because both blood loss and operating time are somewhat less with this technique than with other techniques, further indications would be old age or other medical factors calling for the shortest, rather than the most aesthetically perfect, operation. Occasionally the patient will request it.

Technique

Markings. Accurate and symmetrical markings are most important and are performed with the patient in the upright position prior to induction of anesthesia (I-1). This not only shortens operating time but also avoids the distortion of landmarks which occurs in the supine position.

The midline is marked with a vertical line from the sternal notch through the xiphoid to the umbilicus, as are the midaxes of both breasts from mid clavicle to the nipple. The future nipple location is placed on this latter axis opposite the inframammary fold (I-2). This positioning is checked for both height and symmetry by eye, and more reliably with a tape measure. Each nipple should be from 19 to 21 cm. from the sternal notch, depending on the height of the patient.

The positioning of the anterior skin incision will determine the ultimate size of the breast. Its midpoint will lie on the already marked breast axis, 2 to 3 inches below the future nipple site. From this point it will curve downward, medially and laterally, to meet the inframammary fold at the medial and lateral margins of the breast (I-3, I-4).

The posterior skin incision is performed in the inframammary fold; however, a rounded "tongue," 3 inches across and 2 inches in height, must extend superiorly from the center of the inframammary crease on to the undersurface of the breast (I-5). This flap will provide the ultimate coning of the breast mound when the incisions are closed.

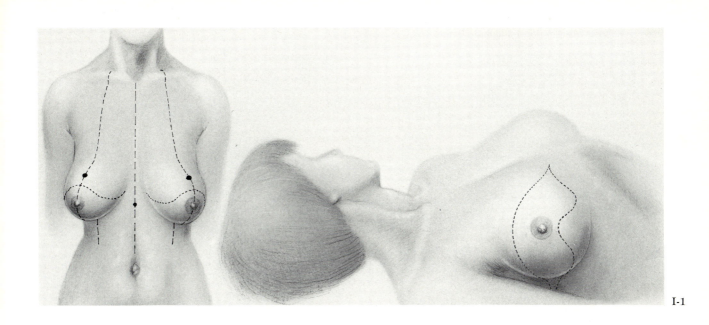

I-1

I-2
I-3

I-4
I-5

55

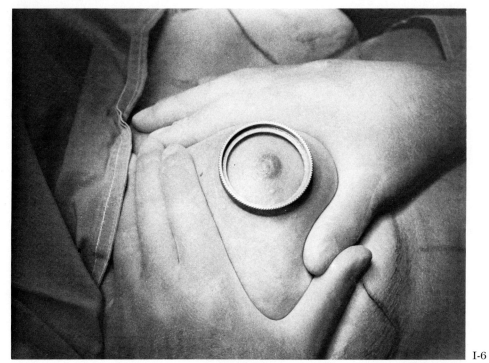

I-6

I-7

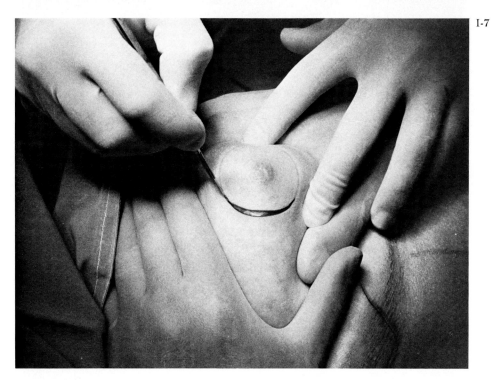

Incisions. The nipple is stretched out by the assistant, and a 5-cm.-diameter circle (outlined by a metal ring) is marked around it (I-6) (almost all nipples of hypertrophic breasts are enlarged and should be reduced to approximately this diameter). The circle is incised (I-7), and the nipple taken as a free full-thickness

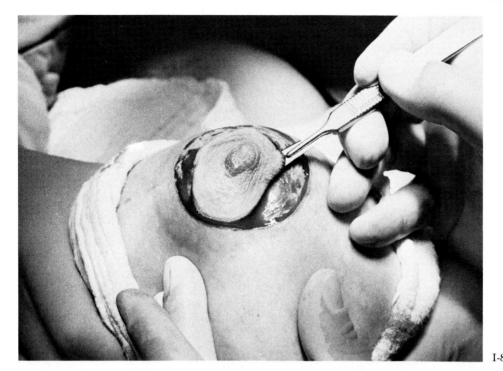

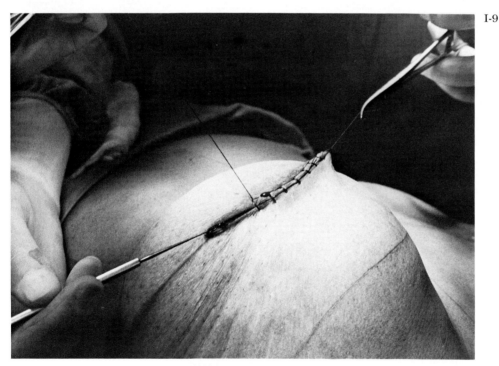

graft (I-8). Bleeding points are cauterized and the defect closed with a hemostatic "whipstitch" (I-9). The nipples are wrapped in a saline sponge and kept in a **safe** place for later placement (even temporary mislaying of the nipples constitutes a true plastic surgical crisis and destroys the harmonious atmosphere of the operating theater).

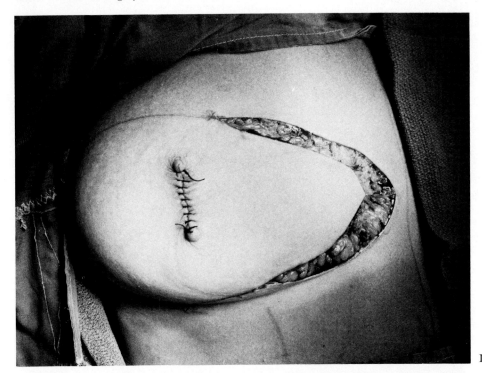

I-10

I-11

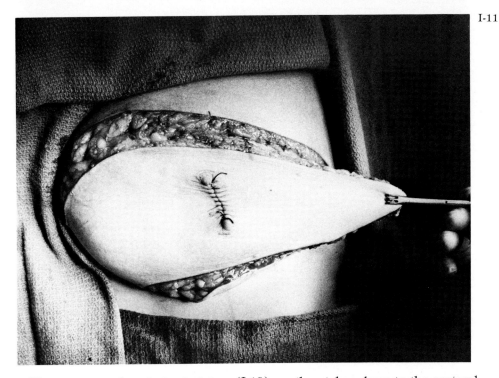

The anterior and posterior incisions (I-10) are then taken down to the pectoral fascia (I-11), using the cutting current of an electric cautery (I-12). All of the breast tissue superior to the anterior incision is left, making the inferior flap about an inch thick (I-13). This effectively removes all the redundant breast tissue; how-

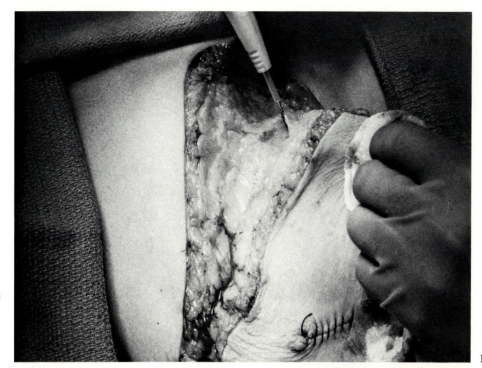

I-12

I-13

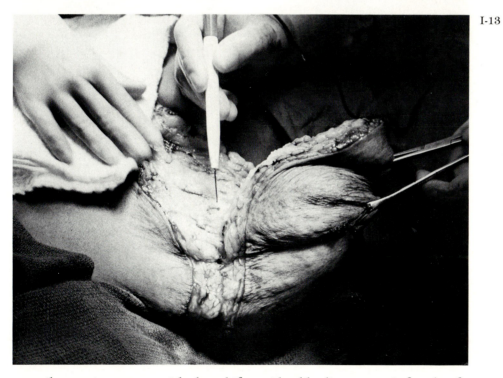

ever, the specimens are weighed, and if considerable discrepancy is found, a further minor resection may be performed on the appropriate side. Hemostasis must be exact during the removal of the breast block because it is during this maneuver that the majority of bleeding occurs.

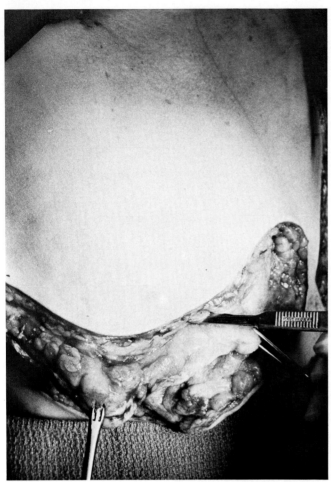

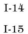

I-14

I-15

Shaping the Residual Breast. The skin edge of the anterior incision is then undermined slightly to allow greater flexibility of the skin (I-14), and a small triangular wedge is taken from the center of the residual upper breast tissue (I-15). This defect is then closed to commence the "coning" of the breast (I-16).

The residual breast tissue, the resultant of an extensive horizontal resection, is then plicated in a vertical fashion to complete the coning and enhance the breast eminence (I-17).

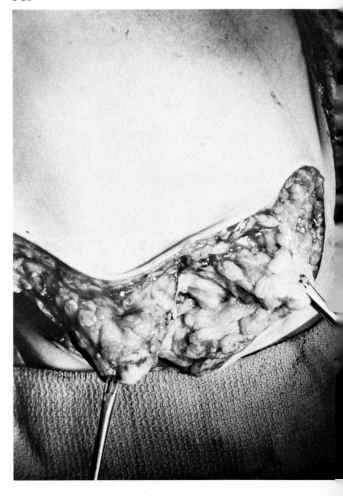

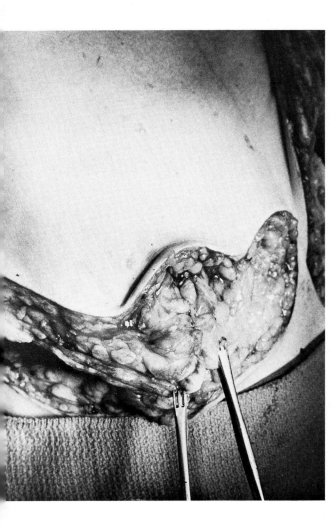

I-16

I-17

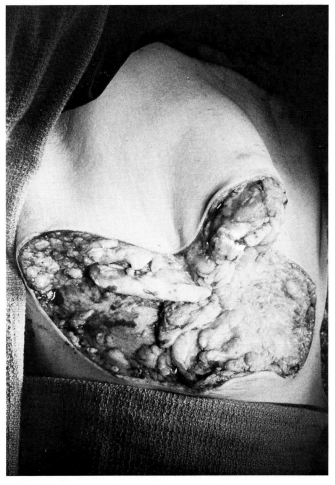

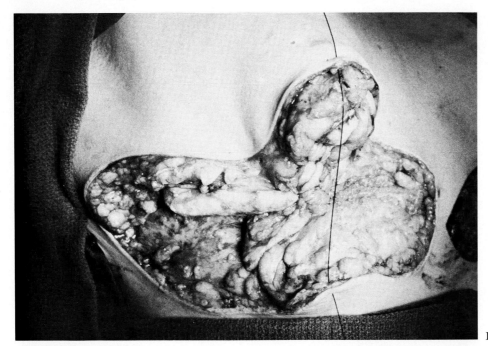

I-18

I-19

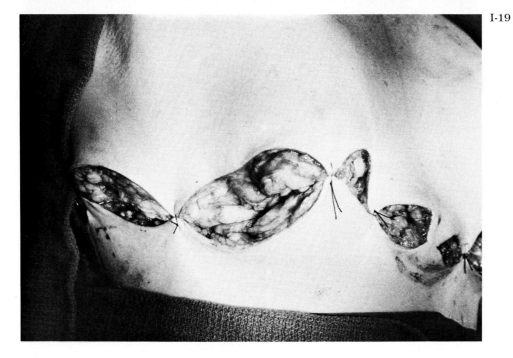

Several temporary stay sutures are placed in the skin (I-18) to judge the plication in terms of ultimate closure and breast shape (I-19). If the breast appears too loose and shapeless, further plication sutures are placed, if necessary fixing the breast to the periosteum of the rib cage. If the result is too tight and "cramped" for a soft, shapely breast, one or more of the plication sutures are removed to allow the breast to assume a more normal shape.

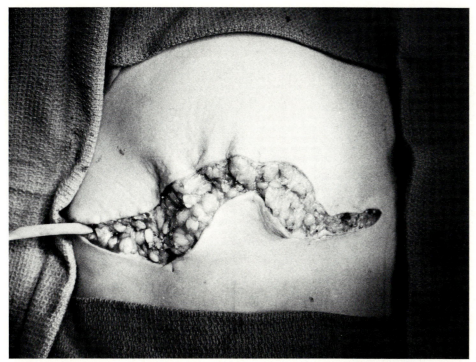

I-20

I-21

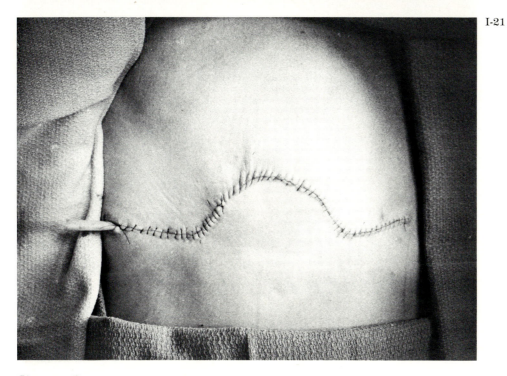

Closure. Closure is accomplished in layers over a soft Penrose drain (I-20, I-21).

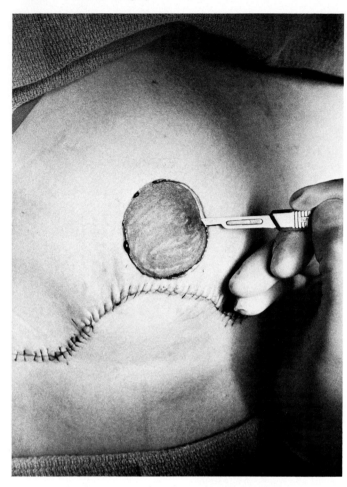
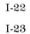

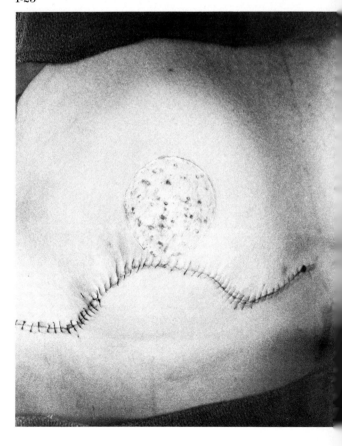

A circular partial-thickness skin graft, 5 cm. in diameter, is taken from the site for the newly located nipple (I-22, I-23). This should lie approximately at the preplanned locus; however, if this appears to be different than the peak of the breast, it is shifted to accommodate the new anatomical situation.

The nipple is carefully sutured on its dermal bed with silk sutures tied and the ends left long (I-24). The edge is adjusted with a running suture of fine nylon (I-25) and the long silk sutures tied over a bolus dressing (I-26).

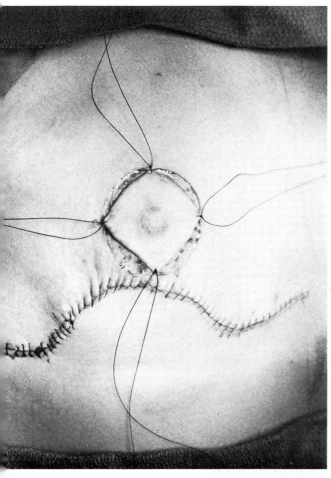

I-24

I-25

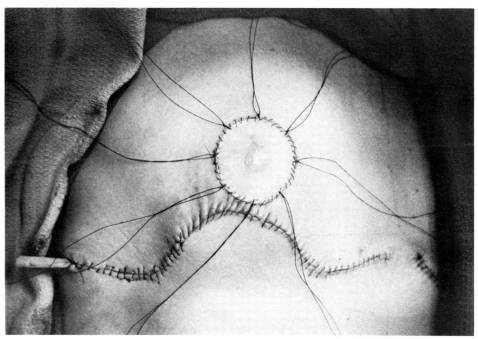

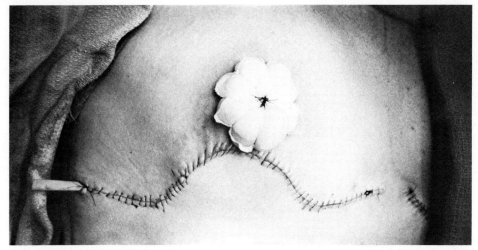

I-26

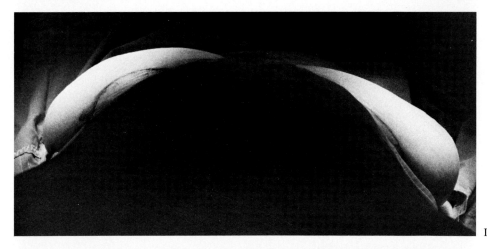

I-27

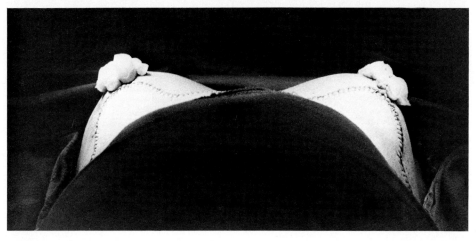

I-28

The patient is placed in a Jobst breast support after conventional drains and dressings are applied.

Pre- and postoperative views of the patient in the supine position are shown (I-27, I-28).

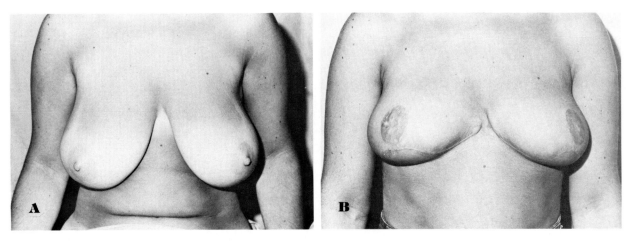

FIG. 3–2.
A. Breast hypertrophy and ptosis preoperatively. B. Following reduction by means of resection and free nipple graft, and showing loss of nipple bulk.

FIG. 3–3.
A. Breast hypertrophy preoperatively. B. Following resection and nipple graft, demonstrating acceptable shape but blurring of the definition of the edge of the nipple.

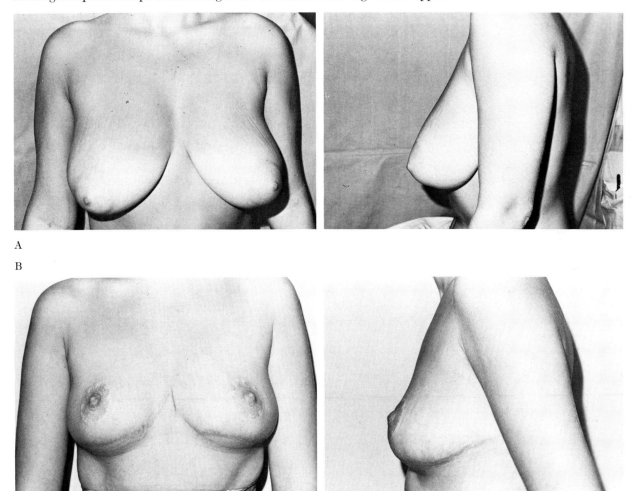

A

B

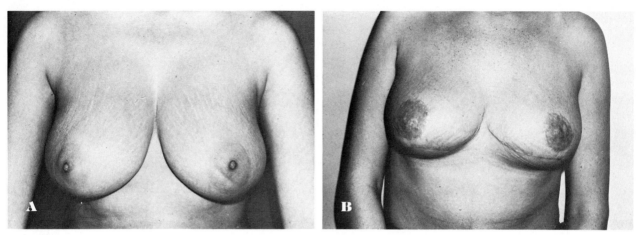

FIG. 3–4.
A. Breast hypertrophy preoperatively. B. An acceptable postoperative result.

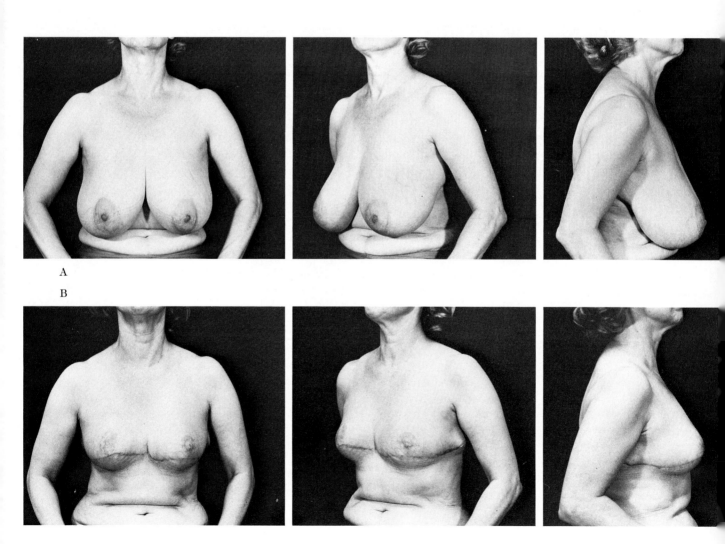

A

B

Representative examples of this procedure, pre- and postoperatively, are shown in Figures 3-2, 3-3, 3-4, and 3-5.

NIPPLE-TRANSPOSITION OPERATIONS

These procedures, in bad repute due to the previously high incidence of vascular complications, have undergone favorable reassessment since the work of Strombeck and are generally regarded as the best procedures where conditions permit, due to the more natural appearance of the healed breast and in particular of the nipple, which is well demarcated from the periareolar skin and usually has unimpaired projection and erectility.

Indications

The indication for a nipple-transposition procedure is whenever reduction of bulk is required, unless the enormity is such as to require the previously described amputation and free-grafted nipple technique, or when other medical considerations dictate a simpler operation with less operating time and less blood loss.

Techniques

Because the resection requires reduction in both the transverse and vertical planes, the planned incisions will generally also be both vertical and horizontal, resulting in an "inverted-T" closure. An alternative technique proposed by Dufourmentel, Mouly, and Schatten employs an oblique lateral wedge. This eliminates the inframammary scar which has a tendency to keloid in its medial portion. This procedure, unsuitable for all except minor breast reductions, is more appropriate to ptosis correction and will be discussed in Chapter 4. All other techniques involve: (1) a "keyhole" incision to reposition the nipple in a superior location; (2) preservation of the nipple on its orthotopic vascular base; and (3) a keel-shaped resection of both skin and breast with an inverted-T closure. The principle variations in these techniques involve different methods of preservation of the in-

tegrity of blood supply to the nipple, since all employ basically similar skin incisions.

In 1960, Strombeck[9] described a procedure based on his vascular studies demonstrating that the principal blood supply to the nipple derived from branches of the lateral thoracic and internal mammary arteries. He resected breast tissue superiorly and inferiorly, leaving the nipple supported on a "bucket-handle" horizontal pedicle of de-epithelialized tissue—the so-called "dermal bridge" (Fig. 3-6).

Although it resulted in a much higher rate of survival of the nipple, this innovative procedure imposed a marked limitation of the degree of reduction obtainable due to the inability to "stuff" lengthy pedicles into a skin envelope of predetermined size. The Strombeck procedure also frequently resulted in somewhat squarish breasts, with nipple retraction being a common problem.

In 1972, McKissock[5] modified the procedure by resecting breast tissue medially and laterally as opposed to superiorly and inferiorly. This left a de-epithelialized vertically oriented bipedicle flap of breast and dermis, including the areola. McKissock states, and this has been confirmed by other authors, that the nipple and areola are more easily elevated, with less tendency to retract. The square flat-bottomed appearance of the breasts was also improved (Fig. 3-7).

Penn[6,7] in a series of papers showed the concept of the "dermal bridge" to be quite fallacious. As long as the circumscribed nipple was supported on a de-epithelialized circle of dermis about 5 cm. greater in diameter than the nipple, it would, unless jeopardized by other hazards, survive. Rather than rely on totally preplanned incisions, he would elevate the nipple into its desired location, resect an appropriate volume of breast tissue inferiorly, tailor the skin envelope to avoid "dog-ears," and place the inferior incision in the submammary fold. This general concept has afforded the author, with modifications described later in the chapter, his best results to date (Fig. 3-8).

◀ **FIG. 3-5.**

A. A major degree of breast hypertrophy, with deep shoulder grooves and a stooped posture. **B.** Following a substantial reduction, marred by prominent and irregular scarring.

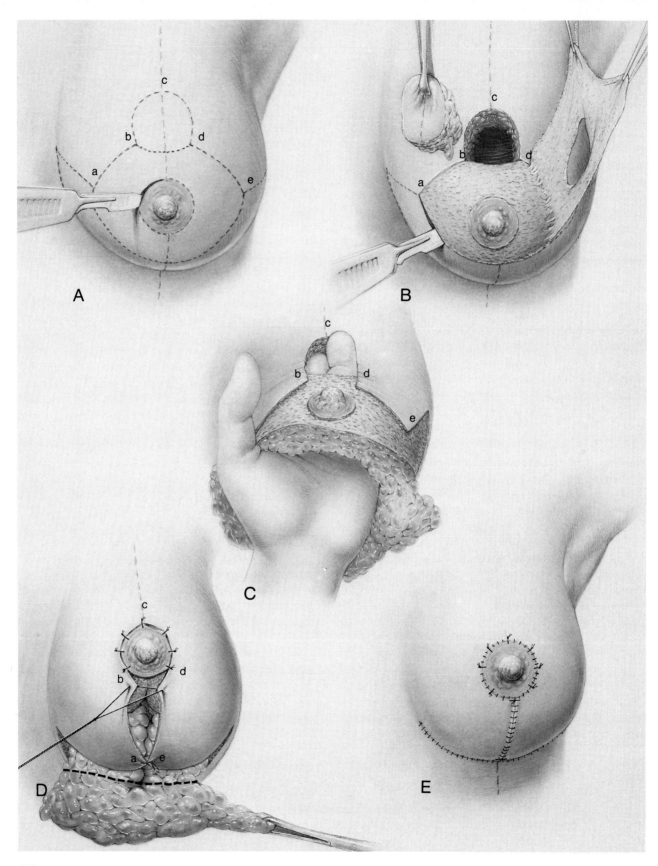

A

B

C

D

E

70

FIG. 3–6.
The Strombeck procedure. Unique features include the preplanned de-epithelialization of a horizontal dermal bridge supporting the nipple. The nipple is elevated into a
space created by resection of a cylinder of skin and breast tissue, and the dermal bridge
◀ is folded under the skin flaps.

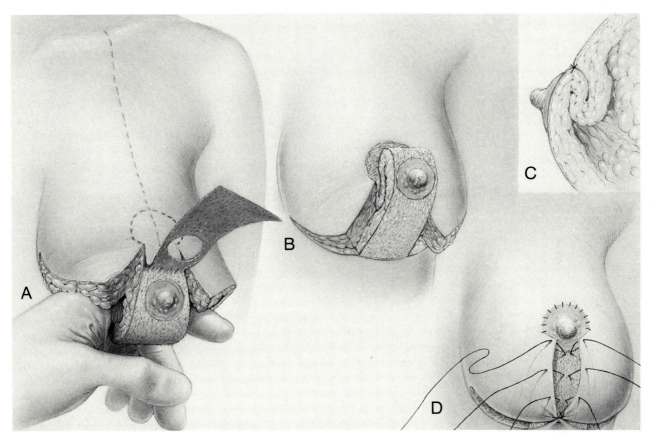

FIG. 3–7.
The McKissock procedure. Resection is planned as with a Strombeck reduction;
however, the dermal bridge is vertically oriented and folded on itself to allow elevation
of the nipple.

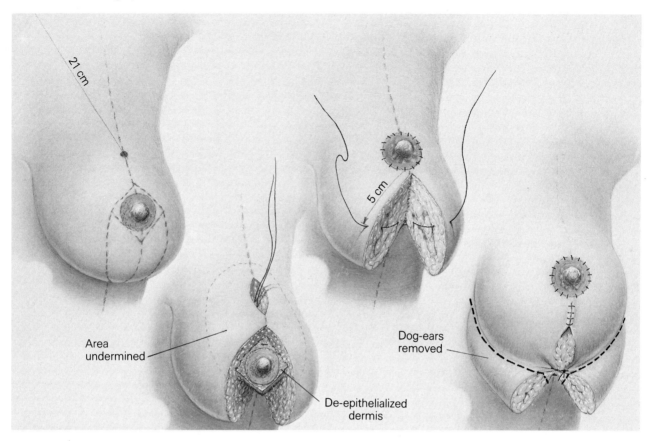

21 cm

5 cm

Area
undermined

De-epithelialized
dermis

Dog-ears
removed

FIG. 3–8.
The Penn procedure, showing the de-epithelialization of
a dermal disk around the nipple, the tightening of the
inferior breast skin, and the freehand elimination of the
dog-ear medially and laterally.

COMPLICATIONS

As with any major resection of tissue in a highly
vascular area, hematoma is an ever-present possibility. Attention to surgical technique and the
placement of soft Penrose drains to allow any
postsurgical oozing to evacuate to the exterior will
minimize the problem. However, if a hematoma of
significant degree is recognized at the first dressing change, it must be evacuated, usually with no
impact upon the ultimate result.

Fat necrosis is both more subtle and more de-
structive. Occurring later than hematoma in the
postoperative course (in many cases after an apparently well-healed operation), it will manifest itself by breakdown of the incision and drainage of
liquified fat for a period of weeks. This complication, unfortunate but unavoidable, may, at worst,
produce asymmetry from loss of bulk or unacceptable puckered scarring, requiring later surgical
revision.

COMPLICATIONS OF RESECTION
AND FREE NIPPLE GRAFT

The procedure itself has certain inherent disadvantages. The planning of the incisions, as described above, with little tension in the vertical
axis, will produce little in the way of "uplift," resulting in a somewhat shapeless breast resem-
bling a sandbag.

The technique of transplanting the nipple as a
free graft will inevitably cause a loss of sensation,
bulk, and erectility, as well as a blurring of definition of the nipple perimeter. Occasionally, partial
or complete slough of the grafted nipple will occur.

For these reasons, most surgeons, including the author, prefer nipple-transposition techniques when technically feasible and medically appropriate. In our current series of nearly 200 breast reductions, only 18 (about 10%) of the procedures have employed the "amputation and nipple graft" technique.

COMPLICATIONS OF NIPPLE-TRANSPOSITION PROCEDURES

Unacceptable aesthetic results, asymmetry, and improper nipple placement (Fig. 3-9) are almost always the result of poor planning. Too much reliance on freehand styling in the recumbent position where landmarks are obscured generally accounts for this error. Therefore, the author feels strongly that marking should always be made in the upright position and, in order to save anesthesia time, prior to induction of anesthesia.

Assuming there has been proper planning, the most frequent complication relates to wound healing and tension. This operation, as many others in plastic surgery, requires a certain degree of tension for its success. An appropriate degree of tension will achieve uplift, but too much will result in wound breakdown (Fig. 3-10).

The vascularity of the skin of the breast may be impaired by an inappropriate choice of procedure or overzealous undermining of skin. There may also be late complications when postoperative edema adds to borderline tension. Fat necrosis is quite common—it is regrettable but unavoidable. Hematoma theoretically is preventable but in practice occurs in between 5 to 10 per cent of these quite massive resections.

Subsequent ptosis is hardly a complication but a recognized sequela of breast reduction. With age, loss of elasticity, and gravity, the condition may recur and will need revision. Rapid weight gain and weight loss are to be avoided because either one will affect the bulk of the breast and, in one way or another, adversely affect the result achieved at surgery.

MANAGEMENT OF COMPLICATIONS

Unsightly scarring caused by prolonged fat necrosis with a sizable fistula eventually healing by contracture, wound breakdown due to excessive tension at the time of closure, or the patient's own tendency to form hypertrophic scars is best man-

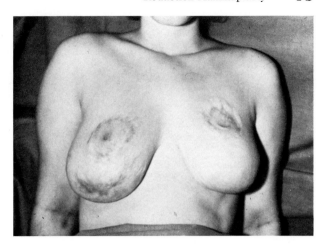

FIG. 3–9.
A grotesquely deformed pair of breasts, showing gross asymmetry, improper nipple positioning, and unacceptable scars. A major challenge for reconstruction.

FIG. 3–10.
Widened scars following wound breakdown, and too great a distance from the nipple to the inframammary fold.

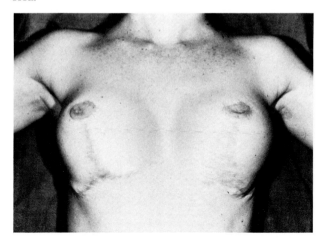

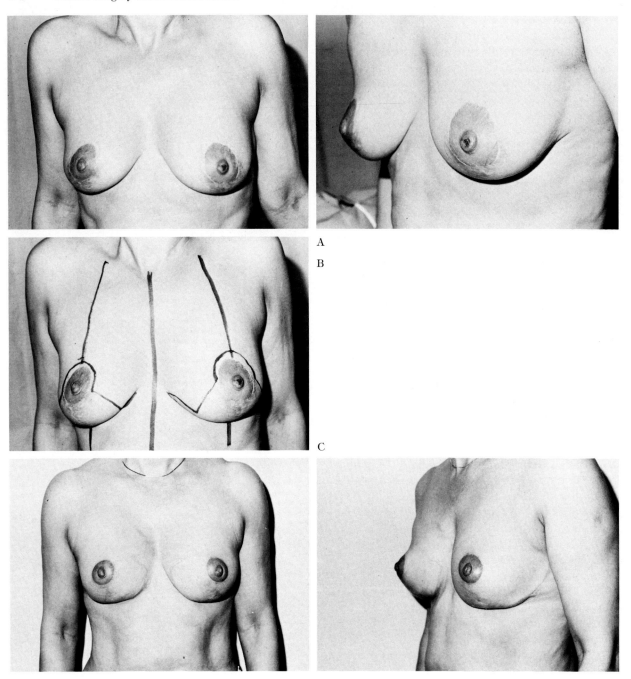

A
B
C

FIG. 3–11.
A. A less dramatic problem than shown in Figures 3-9 and 3-10, but one which demonstrates secondary ptosis, irregular nipples, and widened scars. B. Secondary reconstruction is planned by means of a keyhole resection of excess skin and all of the scar. C. A satisfactory revision with, however, some sacrifice of breast bulk.

aged by simple scar revision with meticulous closure. These revisions are best deferred for at least nine months to a year after the original surgery, in spite of pressure from the patient to alleviate rapidly a distressing situation. Such a time interval will allow the indurated tissue to soften and the adjacent skin to regain elasticity, which will permit closure under less tension than if performed prematurely.

Such complications, though disappointing, are relatively minor and handled fairly straightforwardly. Of far greater consequence, and technically much more demanding, are the distortions resulting from improper planning. Each secondary deformity will have to be assessed individually and managed in such a way that as much symmetry as possible can be gained. Usually this will require a complete "take-down" of the original procedure and careful preplanning of the revision. In most cases, in order to accomplish symmetry, some of the breast size will need to be sacrificed (Fig. 3-11A, B, C).

An important word of caution to the neophyte: if the poor result is due to improper planning in the first place, a revision is vastly more difficult than the initial procedure, and the chances of a happy outcome are slim. Do not be afraid to seek consultation, and humbling though it may be, if necessary turn the case over to a more experienced colleague.

AUTHOR'S CHOICE OF PROCEDURE

When faced with gigantic breasts or excessive ptosis that would preclude the use of nipple-bearing flaps, amputation and free grafting of the nipple is essential. Either the classic Thorek procedure, as described in detail previously in this chapter, or the Strombeck pattern, with block resection of breast tissue and free grafting of the saved nipple onto a de-epithelialized circle at the apex of the resultant cone, may be employed. This operation is, however, always a compromise and gives a less pleasing aesthetic result than nipple-transposition operations.

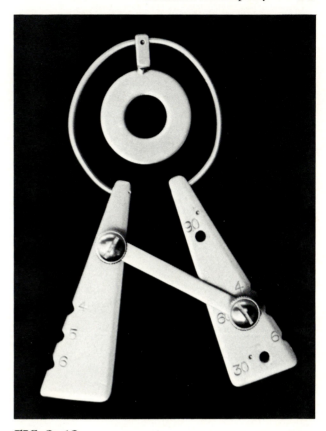

FIG. 3–12.
A prototype of the adjustable metal template for design of the breast reduction incisions.

Whenever possible, a nipple-transposition procedure is employed for the reasons described previously. Although both the Strombeck and McKissock techniques have been used with few complications and with quite uniformly satisfactory results, the author was tremendously impressed by the operation of Penn as demonstrated by Dr. William Powers, who had recently returned from a fellowship in South Africa.

This procedure, with appropriate modifications necessary to suit the preferences of any individual surgeon, yields a happy combination of securely preplanned incisions with a fair amount of leeway for necessary adjustments on the table. The important features are: (1) nipple position and symmetry; and (2) a correct relationship of skin resection and glandular reduction to achieve a pleasing shape appropriate to the patient's body size and the patient's expressed wish, with good "coning" and without undue tension.

MARKING

A flexible wire keyhole-pattern, designed by the author and manufactured by Cosmetech Corporation, is used to outline the site for the new nipple location and to preplan the extent of the skin resection (Fig. 3-12).

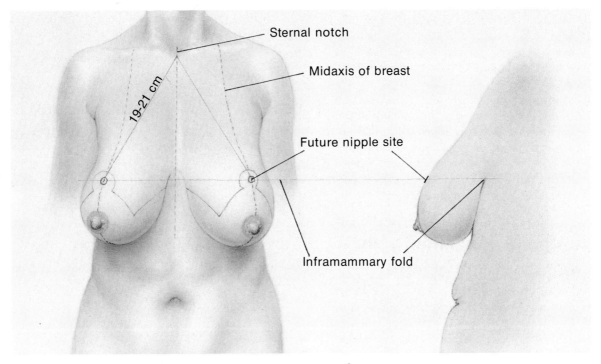

Sternal notch

Midaxis of breast

19-21 cm

Future nipple site

Inframammary fold

II-1

II-2

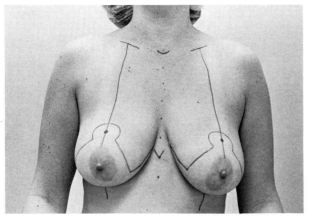

With the patient awake and in the upright position (for reasons explained previously), a line is drawn down the midaxis of the breast from the middle of the clavicle to the top of the existing nipple. A central line is drawn through the sternal notch, the xiphisternum, and the umbilicus. The keyhole is placed so that the top of the new areola will be opposite the center of the inframammary fold in the midaxis of the breast (II-1, II-2).

There are two checks to this positioning: (1) the nipple should lie at the same level as the junction of the middle and distal third of the humerus; and (2) by means of a pendulum on a swing, the distance of the two nipples from the sternal notch should be identical (from 19 to 21 cm., according to the height of the patient).

The keyhole is then spread apart so that its arms can be held at varying angles from each other.

1. A 120° angle will permit a suitable skin resection for a B cup (II-3).
2. A 90° angle will produce a C cup (II-4).
3. A 60° angle, with relatively little skin resection, will allow for a skin envelope representing a D cup (II-5).

The length of the "arm of the keyhole" (the ultimate vertical portion of the incision) may be varied also according to the desired cup size. An arm 4 cm. long will correspond to a B cup; 5 cm. long to a C cup; and 6 cm. long to a D cup.

Markings for the vertical incision should **never** be longer than 6 cm. or the nipple will ride on the upper aspect of the breast, a highly unpleasant aesthetic misjudgment resulting in a very deformed breast. The inframammary fold is marked (also in the upright position) with a small equilateral triangle extending superiorly in the center of this incision. This triangular flap is felt to be extremely important in that it prevents the inherent weakness of a tight "three-point" closure; it can be de-epithelialized to support the closure or modified to adjust the final tension.

The horizontal inframammary incision is initially kept as short as possible both medially and laterally because it can be lengthened toward the end of the procedure to eliminate "dog-ears." Markings for these incisions are joined with a curvilinear line from the end of the arm of the keyhole to the lateral and medial extent of the inframammary incision.

II-3, II-4, II-5

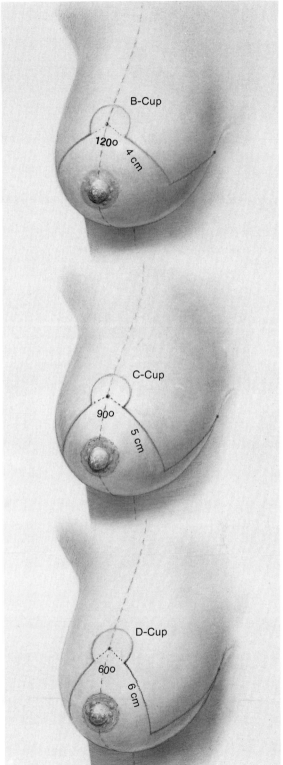

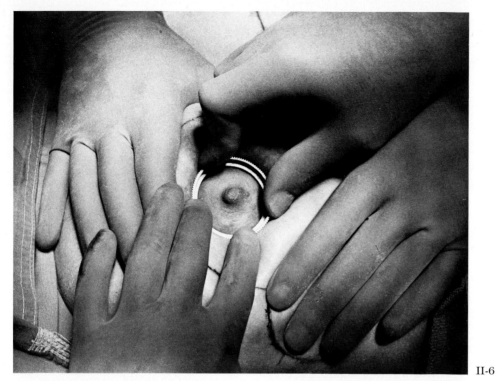

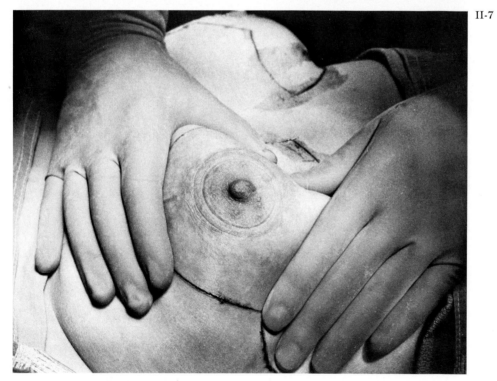

INCISION AND RESECTION

A 5-cm. diameter circle within the areola is centered and marked by means of a metal ring over the nipple eminence (II-6, II-7). This circle is incised into, but not through, the dermis (II-8). The adjacent areolar and skin tissue is de-epi-

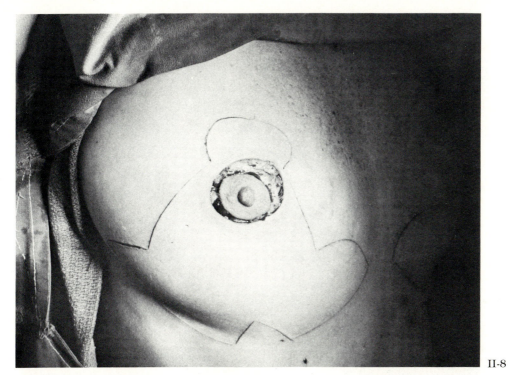

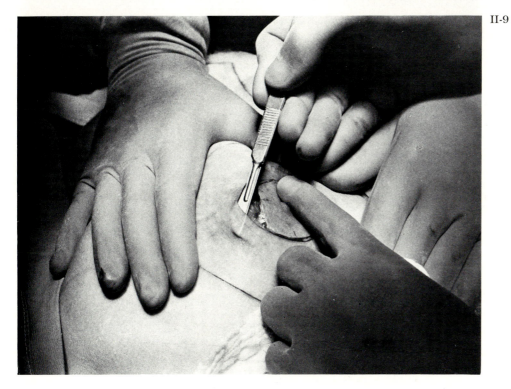

thelialized freehand to a point 3 to 5 cm. beyond the cut nipple edge (II-9). This is all the dermal support that the nipple requires (II-10); beyond this region the skin can be removed down to the fat (II-11).

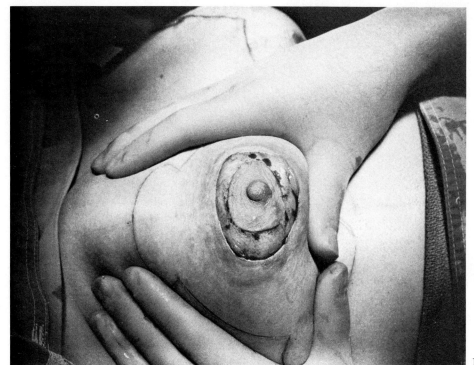

II-10

II-11

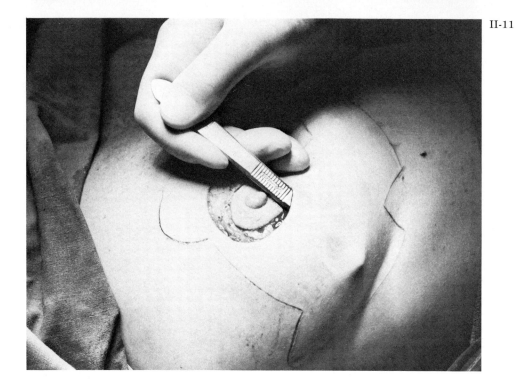

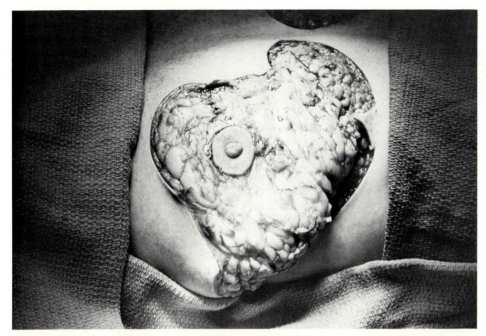

II-12

II-13

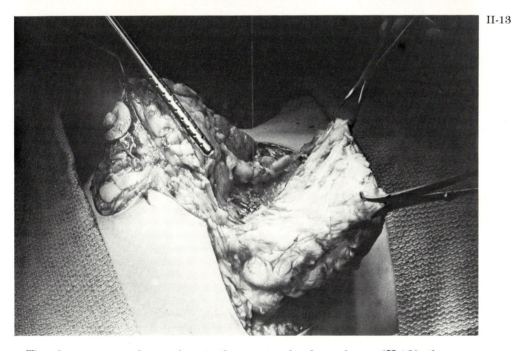

The skin is resected according to the previously planned area (II-12), thus predetermining the size of the skin envelope. From this point on, any modifications in size will depend on the degree of glandular resection. The skin around the circular portion of the "keyhole" is then cautiously undermined and the nipple is elevated into position with two or three stay sutures.

Glandular tissue is then resected (II-13) in a horizontal wedge, the surgeon initially being quite conservative in the amount resected. Skin closure is attempted with stay sutures, and if, as is usual, further glandular resection is required to achieve closure without tension, this is completed.

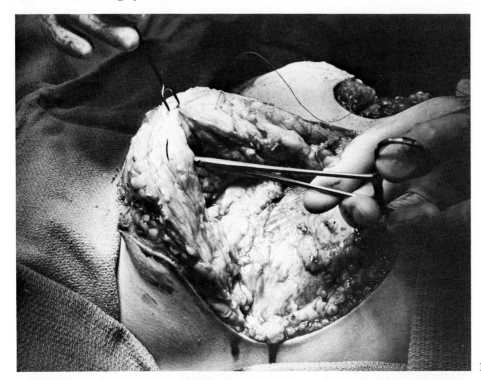

II-14

II-15

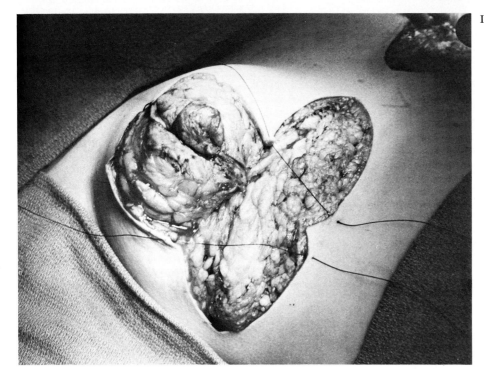

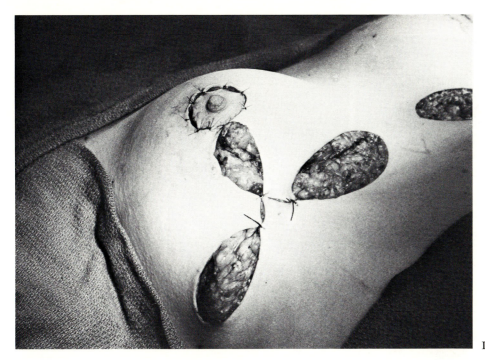

II-16

II-17

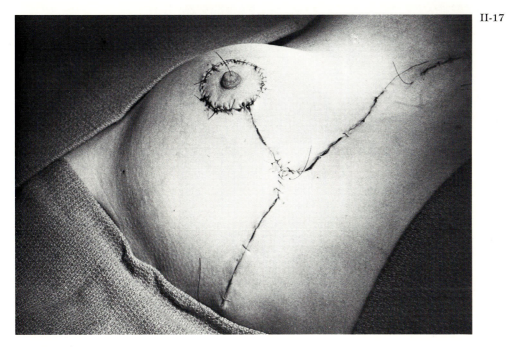

CLOSURE

A careful, layered closure is necessary to minimize scarring. The breast tissue is plicated vertically with heavy chromic sutures (II-14), closing the area resected and achieving a conical shape to the remaining breast tissue (II-15, II-16). After placement of soft Penrose drains, a subcuticular closure is substituted for the stay sutures and Steri-Strips are applied. The inferior triangle may be adjusted to vary the tension. The nipple is positioned with a running suture of fine nylon (II-17), and after applying a conventional fluff gauze dressing a Frederick's-Jobst breast support is applied.

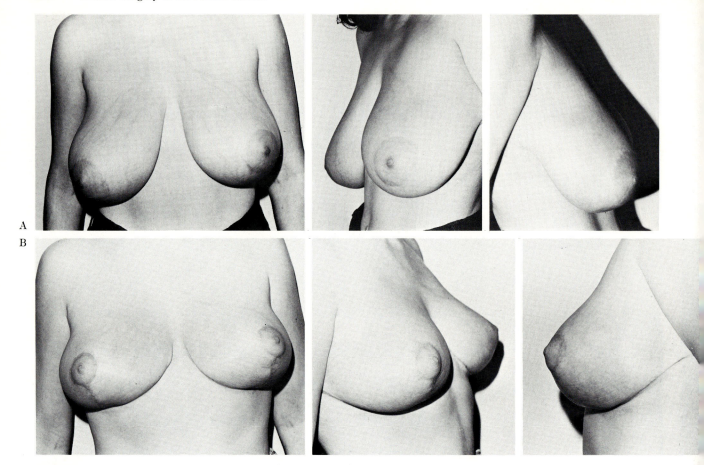

A

B

FIG. 3–14.
A. Breast hypertrophy with moderate ptosis, judged suitable for a nipple-transposition procedure. B. Postoperatively, showing a good conical shape and nipples of near-normal bulk and appearance.

FIG. 3–15.
A. Virginal breast hypertrophy in an adolescent athlete. B. Following a significant re- ▶ duction which yielded an acceptable contour.

FIG. 3–16.
A. Breast hypertrophy, preoperatively. B. Following reduction by the author's method. ▶

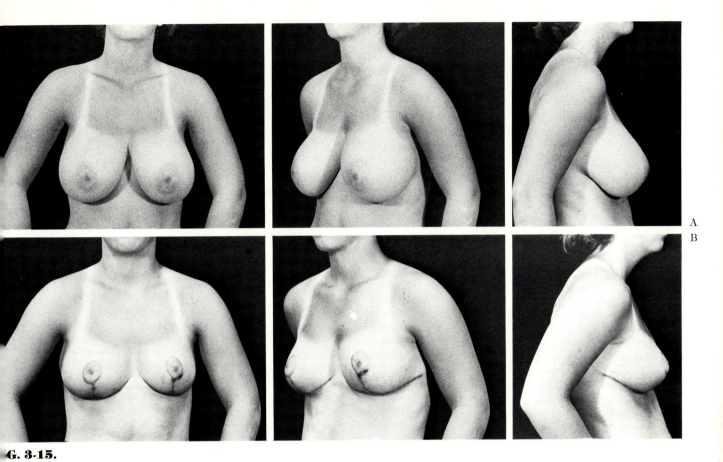

G. 3-15.
G. 3-16.

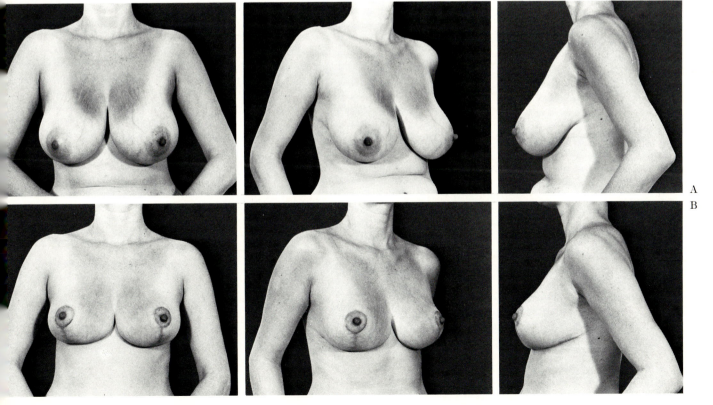

When, however, either the anatomic situation (truly gigantic breasts such that nipple-bearing pedicles would not fit into the skin envelope) or the general medical condition of the patient dictates a simpler procedure, a free nipple graft must be employed. Rather than the Thorek procedure described previously, the author prefers a combination procedure utilizing a keyhole pattern to design the breast resection and a free nipple graft transplanted onto a de-epithelialized recipient site at the apex of the reduced breast.

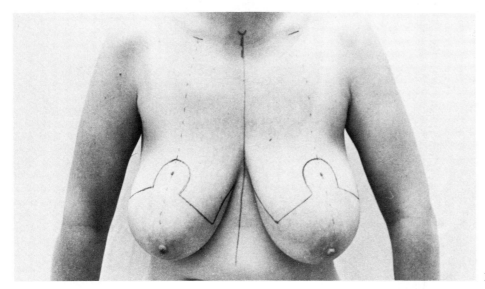

III-1

III-2

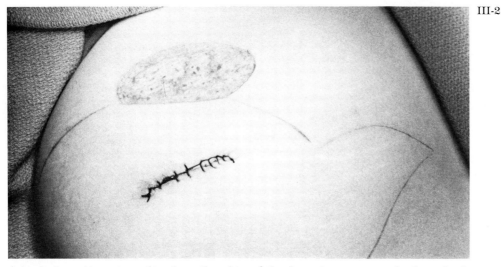

A keyhole pattern is outlined on the skin of the breast as previously described, taking care to position the new nipple site at an appropriate height (III-1). The nipple is resected to a diameter of 5 cm. and preserved for subsequent free grafting. The future nipple site is de-epithelialized (III-2). Resection of the redundant breast tissue proceeds in a block, taking care to incise perpendicularly to the chest wall (III-3). The cutting current of an electrocoagulator is used to prevent excessive blood loss once the skin has been incised (III-4).

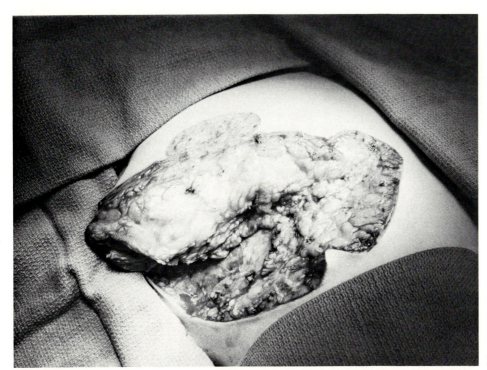

III-3

III-4

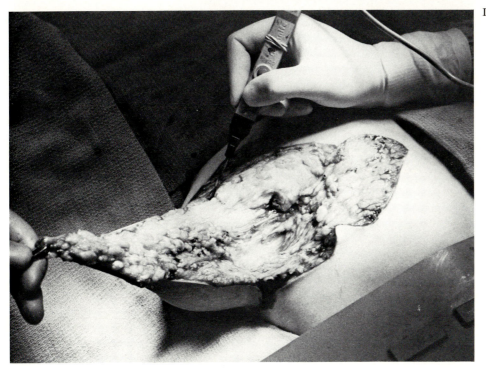

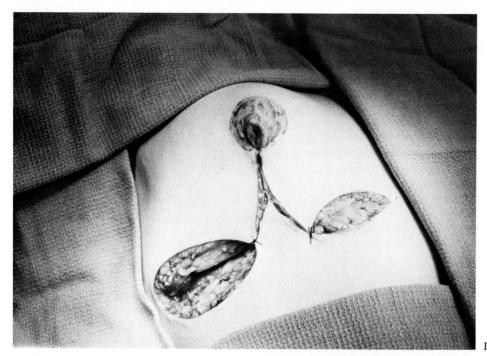

III-5

III-6

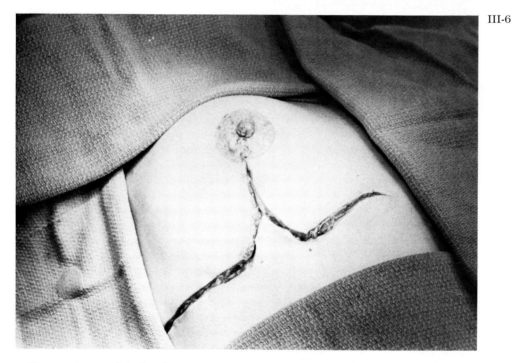

Closure is completed in layers, using stay sutures to test the adequacy of the resection. As can be seen, the de-epithelialized nipple site exhibits a redundancy
(III-5). This redundancy is not trimmed flat, but rather is used to create a central
eminence to the recipient site (III-6). The incisions are closed and the nipple graft
sutured conventionally into place (III-7). The appearance of the breasts in the recumbent position pre- and postoperatively is shown in III-8 and III-9.

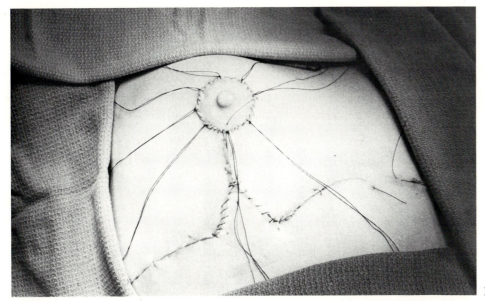

III-7

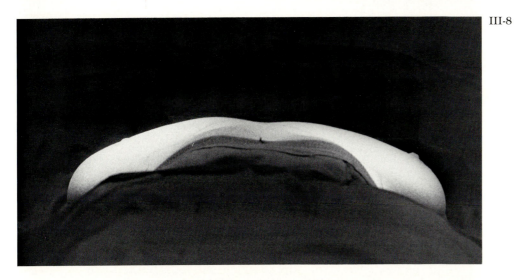

III-8

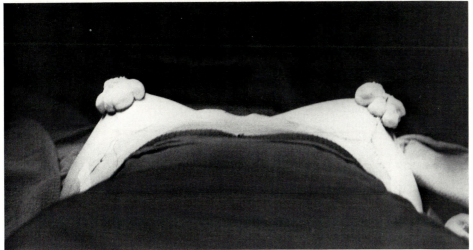

III-9

91

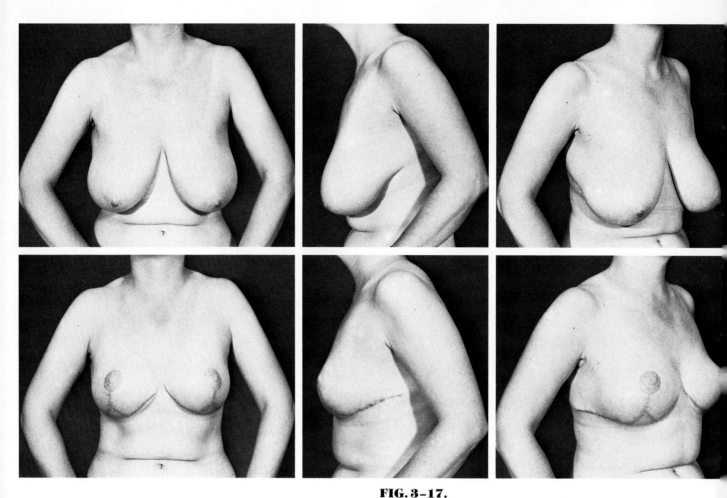

Pre- and postoperative photographs of the patient are shown in Figure 3-17A and B.

As can be seen, the results of this "combination procedure" are considerably more aesthetically satisfactory than those of the more widely used Thorek procedure. However, all of the disadvantages of a nipple graft, rather than a nipple transposition, remain, and use of the combination pro-

FIG. 3–17.
A. Preoperative views of the patient in the preceding surgical sequence. B. The patient 6 weeks postoperative, with well-healed free nipple grafts, prominent early scars, and a satisfactory contour.

cedure should probably be limited to those cases in which a nipple transposition would be, for various reasons previously outlined, unsuitable.

REFERENCES

1. **Biesenberger H:** Deformitaten und Kosmetische Operationen der Weiblichen Brust. Vienna, Maudrich, 1931
2. **Conway H, Smith J:** Breast plastic surgery: reduction mammaplasty, mastopexy, augmentation mammaplasty and mammary construction. Plast Reconstr Surg 21:8, 1958
3. **Joseph J:** Zur Operation der hypertrophischen Hangebrust. Deutsch Med Wochenschr 51:1103, 1925
4. **Lexer E:** Die Gesamte Wiederhertzstellungs—Chirurgie. Leipzig, Barth, 1931
5. **McKissock PK:** Reduction mammaplasty: the vertical dermal flap. Plast Reconstr Surg 49:245, 1972
6. **Penn J:** Breast reduction. Br J Plast Surg 7:357, 1955
7. **Penn J:** Breast Reduction, Trans II. London, International Society of Plastic Surgery, 1960, p 502
8. **Serafin D:** In Giorgiade NG (ed): Reconstructive Breast Surgery. St Louis, Mosby, 1976, p 1
9. **Strombeck JO:** Mammaplasty: report of a new technique based on the two-pedicle procedure. Br J Plast Surg 13: 79, 1960
10. **Thorek M:** Possibilities in the reconstruction of the human form. NY Med J Rec 116:572, 1922

4

correction of breast ptosis and breast asymmetry

BREAST PTOSIS

Ptosis, or drooping, of the female breast is eventually an almost universal condition. It may appear in early adulthood, usually following childbirth and protracted periods of breastfeeding, but more commonly it is an inevitable concomitant of middle age. It is this latter situation that causes most women to seek surgical correction—an otherwise youthful figure is marred by breast ptosis, making the selection and wearing of clothes such as bathing suits and evening dresses awkward and embarrassing.

Ptosis generally results from a combination of two factors:

1. A loss of elasticity in the dermis of the breast skin due either to age or to the continued insult of repeated engorgement and regression accompanying lactation
2. A loss of breast bulk either from postpartum atrophy, age, or rapid weight loss

Ptosis is classified according to the degree of severity, with or without loss of tissue; the aim of surgery is to restore a youthful uplifted contour, and to add bulk if necessary.

HISTORIC ASPECTS

These closely parallel those of reduction mammaplasty and need not be repeated in this chapter.

CONTEMPORARY PROCEDURES

Ptosis correction is generally achieved by resection of excess skin (tightening of the "skin brassiere"), upward transposition of the nipple to a more appropriate position, and plication of the substance of the breast to produce more anterior projection of the breast.

Any of the previously described "nipple-transposition" procedures (see Chap. 3) may be used, including those originated by Dufourmentel,[1] Strombeck,[6] McKissock,[3] Penn,[5] or the author.

Because the Dufourmentel operation, although not the author's personal choice, lends itself to an elegant correction of ptosis, it will be described briefly.

DUFOURMENTEL-MOULY PROCEDURE

Markings are performed in the upright position and involve two initial points of reference (Fig. 4-1A). The eventual nipple position is predicted in the same manner as in other procedures and marked on the breast skin (point a in Fig. 4-1A). A point where the inframammary fold intersects the anterior axillary crease is marked (point b in Fig. 4-1A). The line between these two points represents the axis of the oblique ellipse of skin to be resected.

The width of this ellipse, which will vary from patient to patient, is judged by moving the breast medially (Fig. 4-1B) and laterally (Fig. 4-1C) to determine at what point the skin will close with optimal tension. Excision of skin begins superiorly in an intradermal plane to preserve the dermal blood supply to the nipple. When the nipple has been isolated, skin resection can proceed full thickness laterally and inferiorly until the oblique skin ellipse, excluding the circumscribed nipple, has been removed (Fig. 4-1D).

The skin medial and superior to the resection is undermined and the nipple moved up to its intended position. The ptotic breast tissue is then plicated to itself until adequate "coning" has been achieved, following which the skin ellipse is closed (Fig. 4-1E).

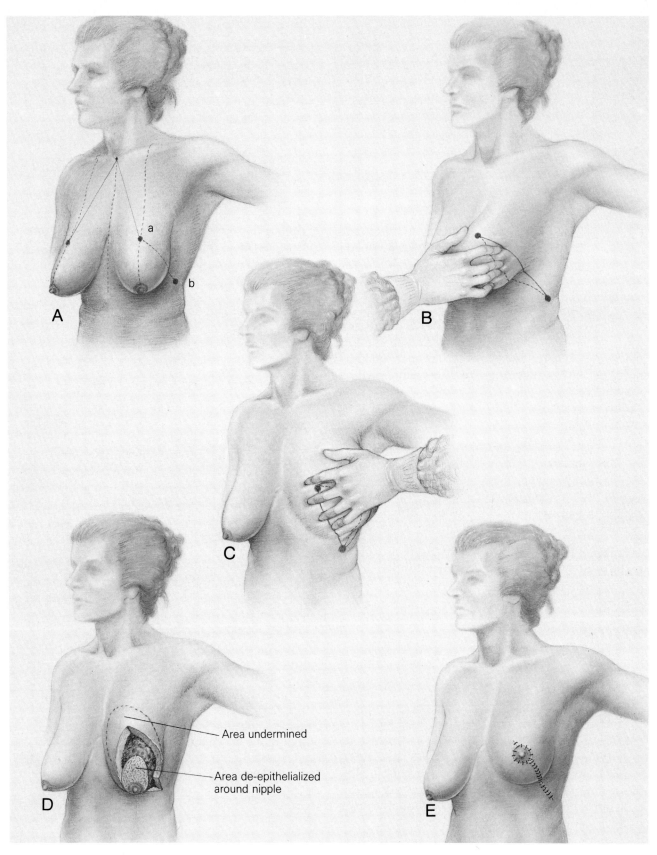

Area undermined

Area de-epithelialized
around nipple

96

FIG. 4–1.
The Dufourmentel procedure. The future nipple site **(a)** is selected, as is a point **(b)** where the inframammary fold intersects the anterior axillary fold. A line is drawn between these two reference points **(A).** The breast is then pulled medially **(B)** and laterally **(C)** to define the skin resection **(D).** The nipple on a vascular dermal disk is moved into position, the breast tissue plicated, and the ◄ skin closed **(E).**

FIG. 4–2.
Markings for a secondary ptosis correction with elevation of the nipple and revision of previous scars.

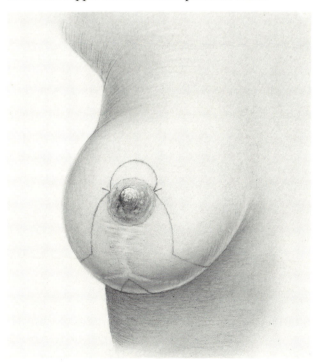

This procedure is held in wide regard, particularly in Europe, but has, in the author's limited experience, certain significant drawbacks.

1. The scar often extends inferiorly and laterally on the chest wall beyond the confines of a brassiere or the upper half of a two-piece bathing suit.

2. There is a tendency to place the nipples too high and too medially—the "upward squint." The author has seen several unfortunate examples of this in his practice, a secondary deformity which is most difficult to correct.

3. Even though the immediate result may be impressive, the design of the operation is such that the distance between the inferior margin of the nipple and the inframammary crease is greater than ideal. In later years the breast will tend to sag.

4. The rather "freehand" nature of the procedure, where judgment of tension in the recumbent position calls for a high degree of sophistication, makes it an unwise choice for the inexperienced surgeon.

COMPLICATIONS

The principal complication will result, inevitably, from the surgeon's desire to achieve as much correction as possible. The degree of tension on the closure will parallel the "uplift" achieved, and, if exceeded, will endanger wound healing. Dehiscence and delayed healing will therefore be the most frequent complication.

On the other hand, inadequate tension will yield an insufficient correction of the condition, leading to the question "How tight is tight enough?" Strain gauges will not tell us and it must be up to the judgment of the surgeon at the operating table to make this subtle decision. Even though dehiscence is a major inconvenience for the unfortunate individual patient, it is inevitable, given the vagaries of wound healing, that it will occur occasionally in the hands of even the most skillful surgeon.

Capsular contracture, previously described in detail in Chapter 2, may be a complication if an implant has been employed, and is managed as already outlined. Nonoperative capsulotomy (the "breast squeeze") is first attempted; if unsuccessful, an open capsulectomy is performed.

SECONDARY CORRECTION OF BREAST PTOSIS

Secondary ptosis is hardly a complication, but rather a recognized, if unfortunate, possible sequela to any operation designed to correct skin laxity. The underlying cause, loss of tone and elasticity of the skin, is, of course, unaffected by the surgical procedure, and may well permit the condition to recur.

Operative correction will depend upon the existing anatomic situation. The entire breast, nipple and all, may again become ptotic; on the other hand, the nipple may remain in its "correct" location while the breast mass sinks, causing the skin of the lower pole of the breast with its attendant scars to stretch.

In the former situation (and this, of course, is judged by measurement of nipple height and position), a complete reoperation utilizing a keyhole pattern in the appropriate location will be necessary (Fig. 4-2). The results of such a procedure are illustrated well in Chapter 3 (Fig. 3-11A, B, C).

In the latter, and less common, situation, a different approach must be employed without elevation of the nipple. A typical example of this situation is shown in Figure 4-3.

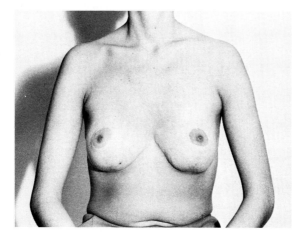
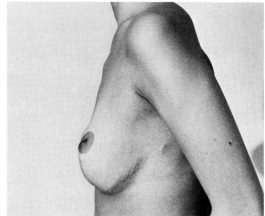

FIG. 4–3.
A typical case of secondary ptosis without displacement of the nipple. Operative Sequence I (steps 1 through 10) illustrates surgical correction.

Incisions are planned so that both a vertical and horizontal wedge of skin will be removed (I-1). The vertical excision starts just below the nipple and includes the old vertical scar (I-2). The horizontal wedge has as its lower border the inframammary fold; the upper margin is placed so that enough skin will be resected to achieve correction without undue tension (I-3).

I-1

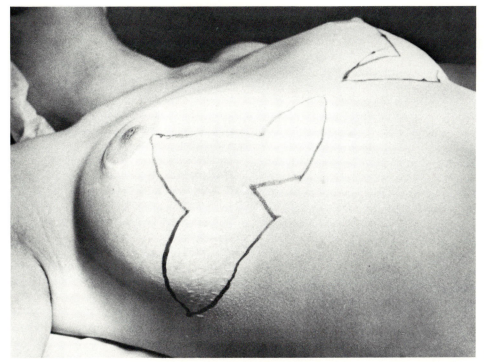

I-2

I-3

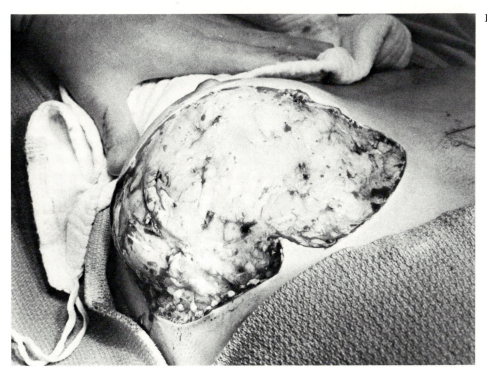

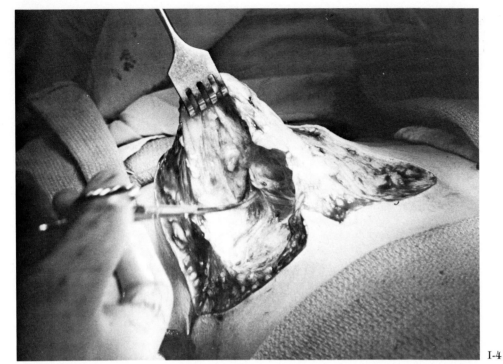

I-4

I-5

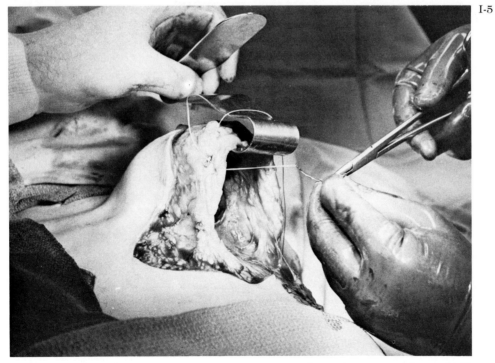

After resection of the skin, the breast is dissected from the pectoral fascia (I-4) to allow a vertical plication (I-5) and coning of the breast tissue itself (I-6). Temporary stay sutures are placed in appropriate locations to test the effectiveness of the correction (I-7).

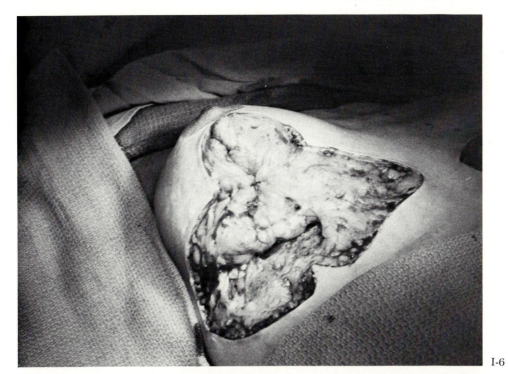

I-6

I-7

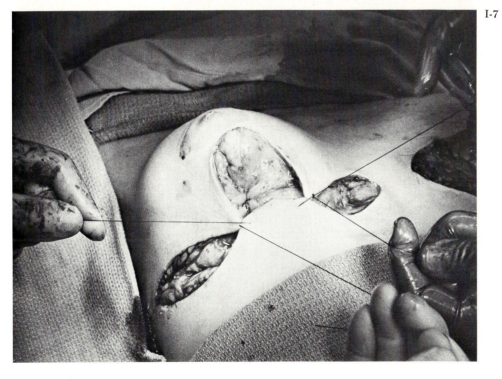

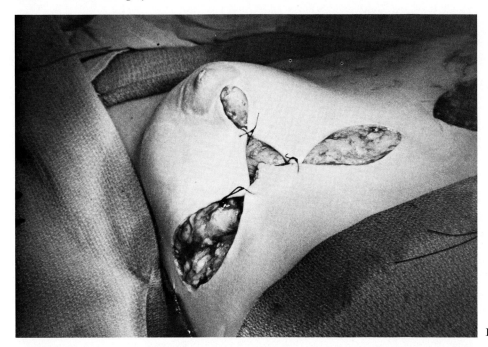

I-8

I-9

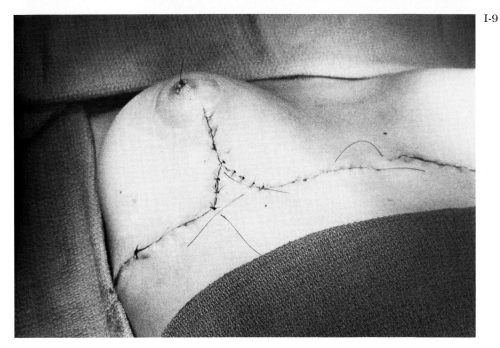

   If too loose, further skin is resected until the closure is tight enough. If the bulk of breast tissue prevents closure without undue tension (a fine point of surgical judgment best determined by blanching of the skin at the location of the stay sutures), some of the breast must be resected (I-8).

   When the correct balance has been achieved, the stay sutures are removed and a layered closure (over a drain, if necessitated by persistent oozing) is completed. The inferior skin triangle may be modified to "fine tune" the tension on the closure (I-9).

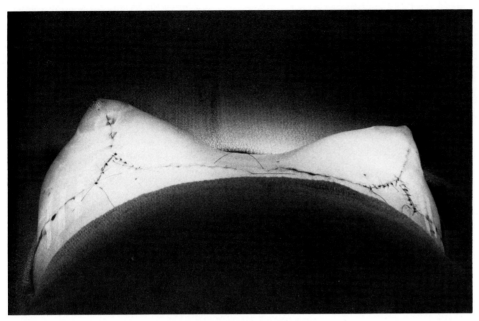

I-10

The postoperative correction achieved by this procedure is shown, in the recumbent position, in I-10. Postoperative management is identical to that of the original ptosis correction or a reduction mammaplasty.

AUTHOR'S CHOICE OF PROCEDURE

The operation must be chosen very carefully to suit both the existing anatomic situation and the patient's expressed desire for a specific result. The basic operative technique must be varied according to the classification of the ptosis and the exact existing anatomic condition. There are three broad categories, each requiring its own operative approach.

MILD PTOSIS WITH MAJOR LOSS OF BULK

In a few cases, mostly due to postpartum atrophy, this condition will respond to a simple bilateral augmentation mammaplasty. However, the surgeon must be extremely careful in the selection of these cases and not yield to the temptation of choosing an operation on the basis of its simplicity when the anatomic situation is inappropriate.

If the degree of ptosis is more than "mild," an augmentation will produce an unsightly "double-bubble" contour, with the nipples lying inferior to the apex of the augmented breast mound and pointing toward the patient's feet. A good common sense rule is **never** to simply augment when the nipples, in the upright position, lie below the inframammary fold. Such cases will always require a tightening of the "skin brassiere."

PTOSIS WITH ADEQUATE BREAST TISSUE

This is the most common situation, and can be adequately corrected by any of the previously described nipple-transposition procedures (see Chap. 3), except that the resection of glandular tissue is eliminated. The author prefers his own modification of the Penn technique, because he feels that the inferiorly displaced nipple can be safely moved a greater distance without the limiting factor of discrete flaps which have to be folded within a markedly reduced skin envelope.

This has already been described in detail; however, the significant points in planning and execution deserve reemphasis.

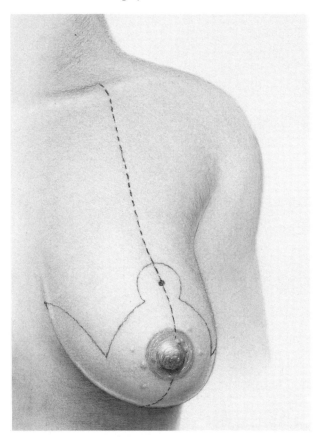

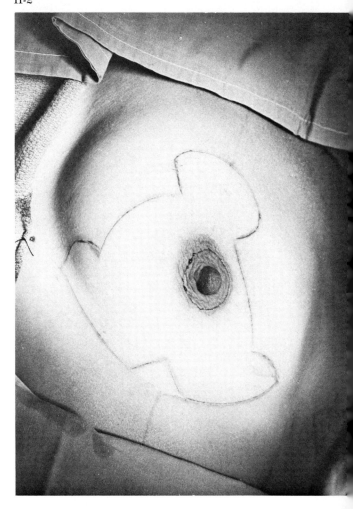

1. The desired nipple location is plotted in the upright position (II-1), and, using this point for placement, the flexible wire pattern is used to design a keyhole-shaped pattern (II-2) which will establish the amount of skin to be resected (II-3). The inframammary fold will constitute the inferior incision.

2. The glandular portion of the breast is then sharply (II-4) and bluntly (II-5) dissected from the pectoral fascia (II-6) and plicated to itself in a vertical fashion to achieve "coning" of the breast (II-7). It may also be fixed to the chest wall to reduce tension on the skin closure.

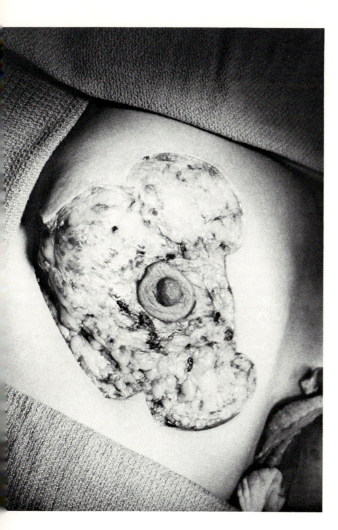

II-3

II-4

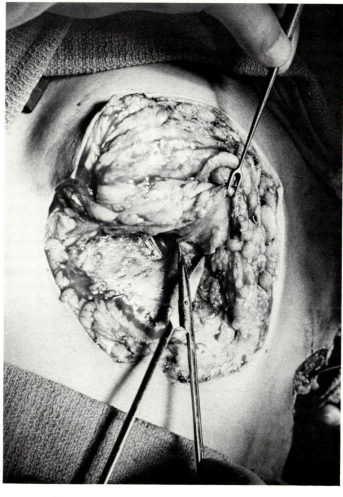

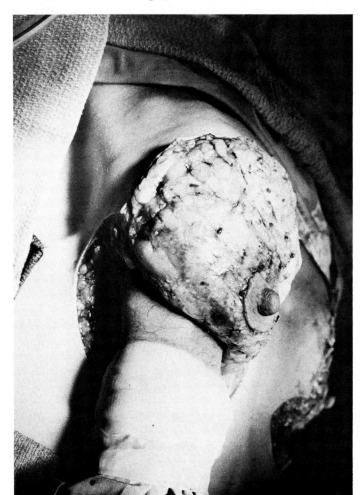

II-5

II-6

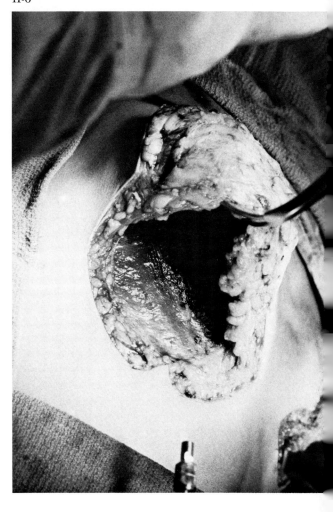

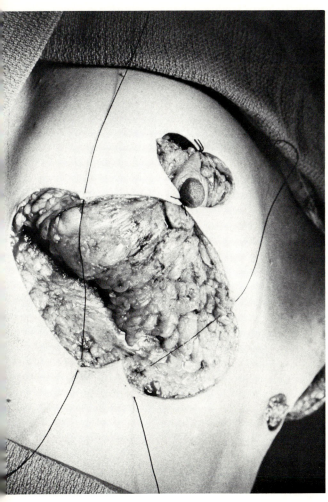

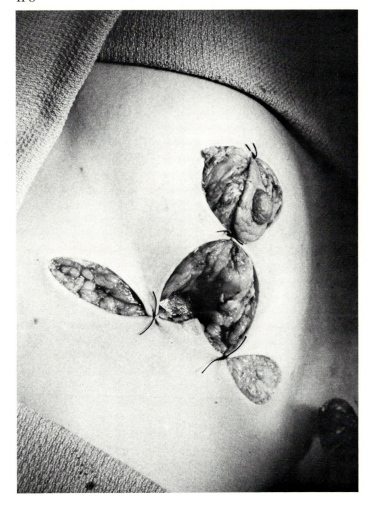

3. The circumscribed nipple, on its de-epithelialized dermal base, is moved into position and the skin closed under as much tension as will produce adequate uplift without endangering wound healing (II-8).

4. If, upon closure, it is evident that a slight misjudgment has been made, the situation can and must be corrected "on the table." If the closure is too loose, further skin may be resected from the edges of the vertical suture line running from the nipple to the inframammary fold. If, on the other hand, closure can only be achieved under extreme tension (II-9), breast tissue must be resected (II-10) in as much quantity as necessary to reduce the pressure on the skin edges (II-11).

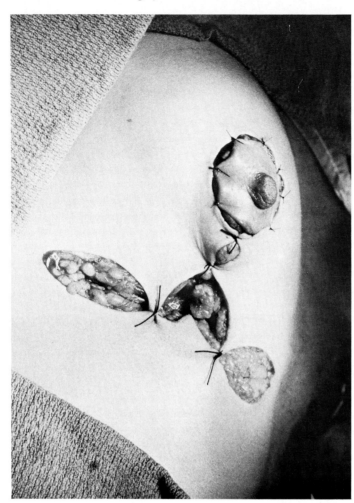

II-9

II-10

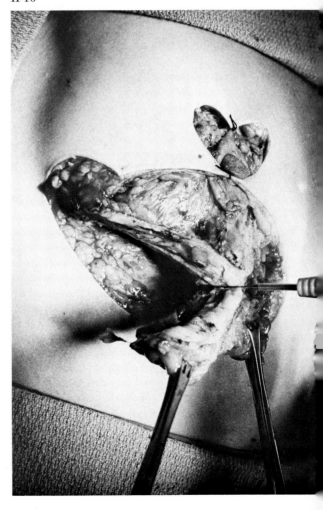

II-11

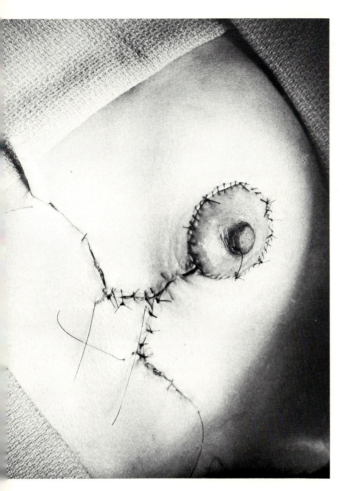

MODERATE TO SEVERE PTOSIS WITH LOSS OF BULK

This condition may require, in addition to mamma-pexy as described, an addition of bulk by means of a prosthesis.

III-1

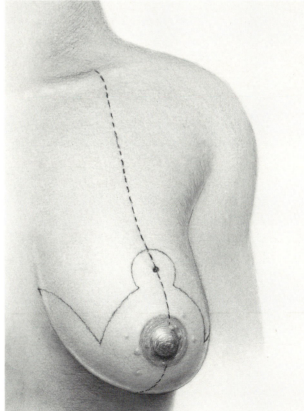

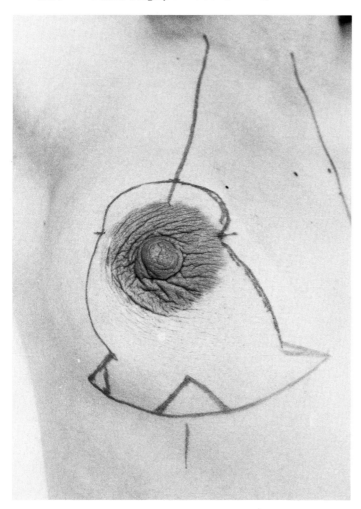

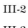

III-2

III-3

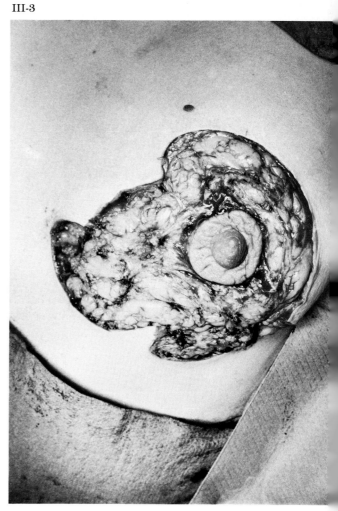

First the skin is resected (III-1, III-2, III-3) and nipple repositioning (III-4) and plication of breast tissue to itself (III-5) are accomplished.

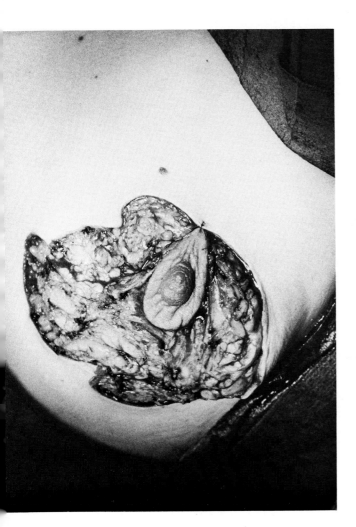

III-4

III-5

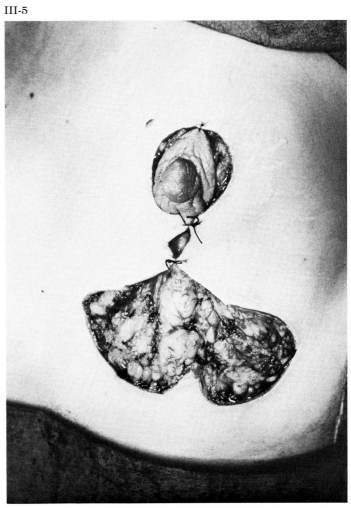

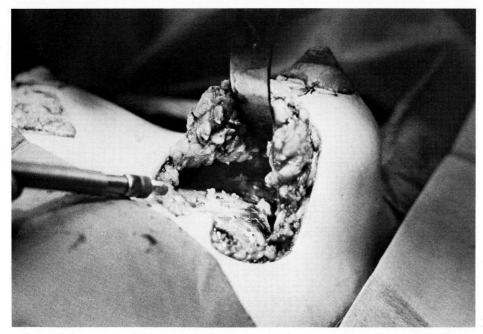

III-6

III-7

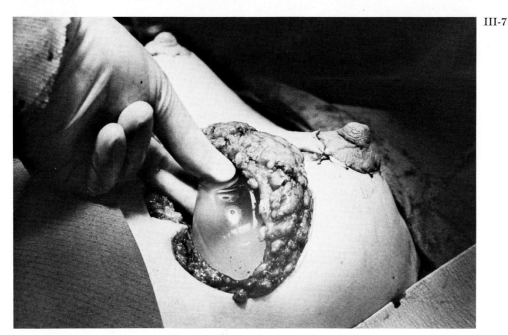

A retromammary pocket is dissected at the level of pectoral fascia (III-6) and an implant is inserted into this location (III-7) (this procedure is uniquely suited to the inflatable type of implant rather than the implant of fixed size).

Closure of the skin is tested with stay sutures (III-8), and the implant is replaced with one of different size if necessary.

When the appropriate size and contour are achieved, closure is completed as previously described (III-9). The condition supine at the end of the procedure is shown in the last photograph of the sequence (III-10). Another typical result is represented by Figure 4-4A and B.

Activity is limited just as for any augmentation mammaplasty in an attempt to avoid capsular contracture.

112

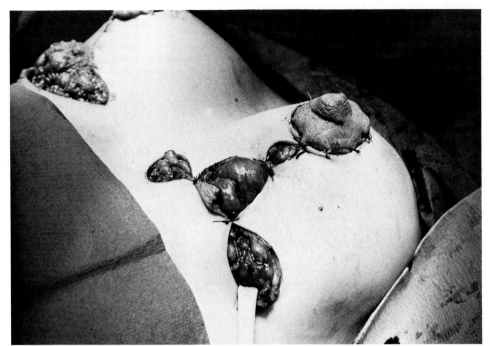

III-8

III-9

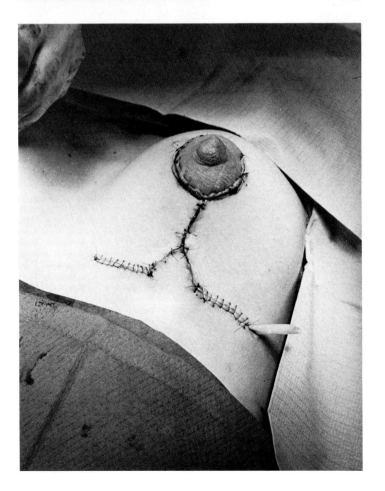

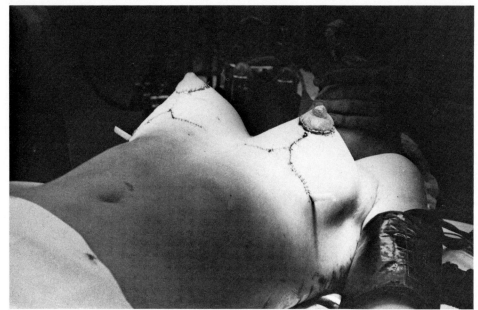

III-10

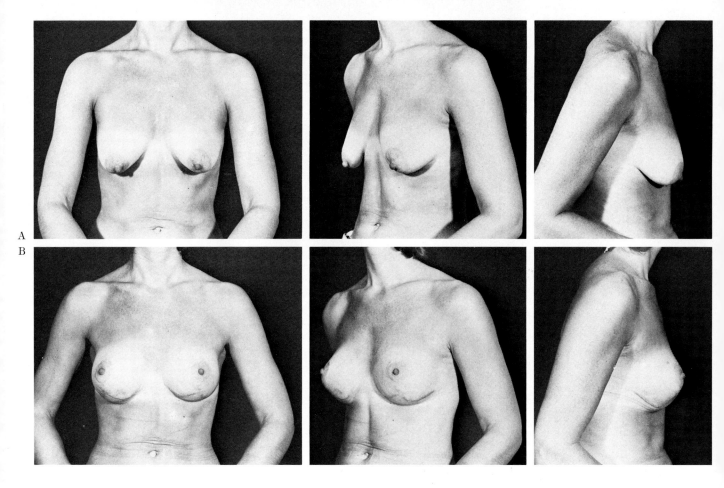

A

B

◀ **FIG. 4–4.**
Correction of ptosis with loss of bulk by means of simultaneous breast elevation and prosthetic augmentation A. Preoperative condition. B. Corrected situation.

FIG. 4–5.
Correction of major ptosis with loss of bulk in two stages. A. Preoperative situation. B. Following ptosis correction only. C. After prosthetic augmentation three months later.

This combined procedure is best reserved for those surgeons emotionally equipped to handle the tension (both psychological and that related to wound healing) involved. A combination mammapexy and later augmentation can always be done in two stages, with the advantage of greater security and the disadvantage of extra morbidity and expense to the patient. Such a case is illustrated by Figure 4-5A, B, and C.

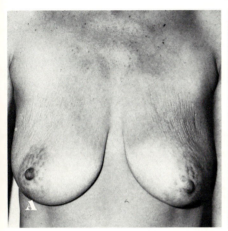 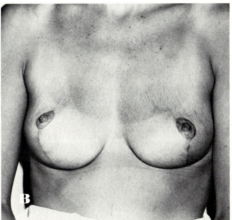 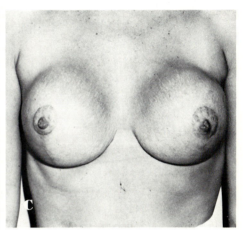

BREAST ASYMMETRY

Breast asymmetry, which we are seeing with increasing frequency in our practice, is one of the most fascinating areas of breast reconstruction. It is, in a wry way, encouraging to see youngsters presenting with this psychologically devastating condition at an age when they can be rehabilitated surgically; it is also a healthy reflection of the useful dissemination of information about what the specialty of reconstructive surgery can achieve.

Breast asymmetry presents itself in such myriad forms that it almost defies classification,[2] and its successful correction demands not only the highest standards of surgical expertise but also an aesthetic appreciation which befits the sculptor rather than the surgical artisan. A gross classification could be summarized as follows:

Unilateral hypomastia
Unilateral hypermastia
Combination of both
Asymmetric hypomastia
Asymmetric hypermastia

HISTORIC ASPECTS

Very little has been written about breast asymmetry other than about a small series of individual cases. Historically, no trends or philosophies are seen emerging.

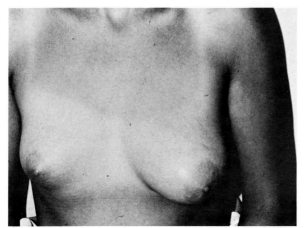

A

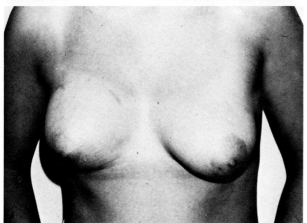

B

FIG. 4–6.
Unilateral hypomastia (A) corrected by unilateral augmentation (B).

FIG. 4–7.
Unilateral hypomastia (A) corrected by augmentation of the hypoplastic side and elevation of the "normal" side (B).

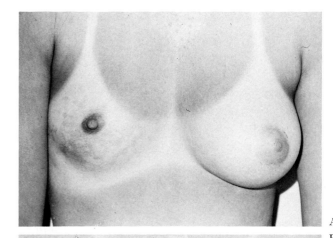

A

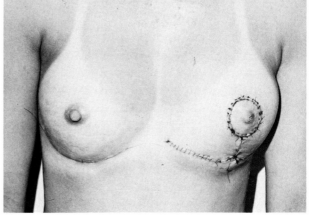

B

CONTEMPORARY PROCEDURES

Again very few trends are dominant: each case is dealt with on a very individual basis, using as a basic guideline the classification given above. It must be stressed that these groupings are somewhat arbitrary, and a high degree of surgical and judgmental sophistication must be applied to each individual case in order to obtain an optimal result.

UNILATERAL HYPOMASTIA

This may range from a mild discrepancy in size between the affected breast and its normal sister organ, to Poland's syndrome[7] which includes breast and nipple agenesis, absence of the pectoral musculature, and abnormalities of the rib cage on the involved side. Rarely will a simple unilateral augmentation suffice (Fig. 4-6A, B). Due to the difficulty in matching a normal structure, it is usually

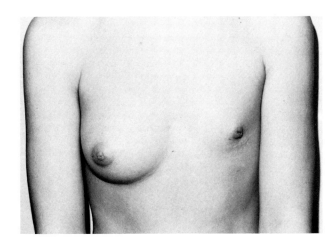

FIG. 4–8.
Poland's syndrome with breast agenesis and anomalies of ribs and pectoral muscles.

necessary to modify the opposite breast either by means of an augmentation of lesser degree or a mammapexy to elevate the normal breast when it is slightly ptotic (Fig. 4-7A, B).

Poland's syndrome requires a custom-built prosthesis with a superior extension to fill in the infraclavicular hollow caused by absence of pectoral musculature (Fig. 4-8). A new and elaborate procedure, the latissimus dorsi flap,[4] will, in conjunction with an augmentation, provide an even better contour (see Chap. 6).

UNILATERAL HYPERMASTIA

Again, only rarely and with unusual anatomy will it be possible to achieve symmetry with a unilateral reduction mammaplasty. It will almost always be necessary to operate on both sides, even though one side is apparently normal (Fig. 4-9A, B).

One of the great advantages of a template, or a flexible wire pattern such as that designed by the author, is that it preplans symmetrical incisions even though the amount of skin to be resected is unequal. In this way it is possible to correct discrepancies in bulk or contour and arrive at a symmetric end-point.

In most cases, a reduction on the larger side and a ptosis correction on the normal side will produce a symmetric and improved contour.

COMBINATION OF HYPO- AND HYPERMASTIA

This condition is probably the most common one the plastic surgeon has to face, and it is also possibly the most difficult one to deal with. Certainly an

FIG. 4–9.
Unilateral hypermastia (A), treated by reduction mammaplasty with simultaneous elevation of the "normal" side (B).

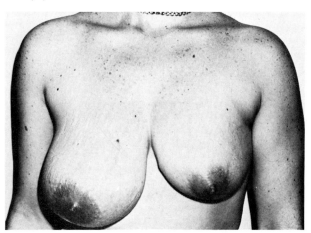

A

B

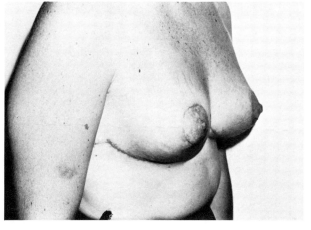

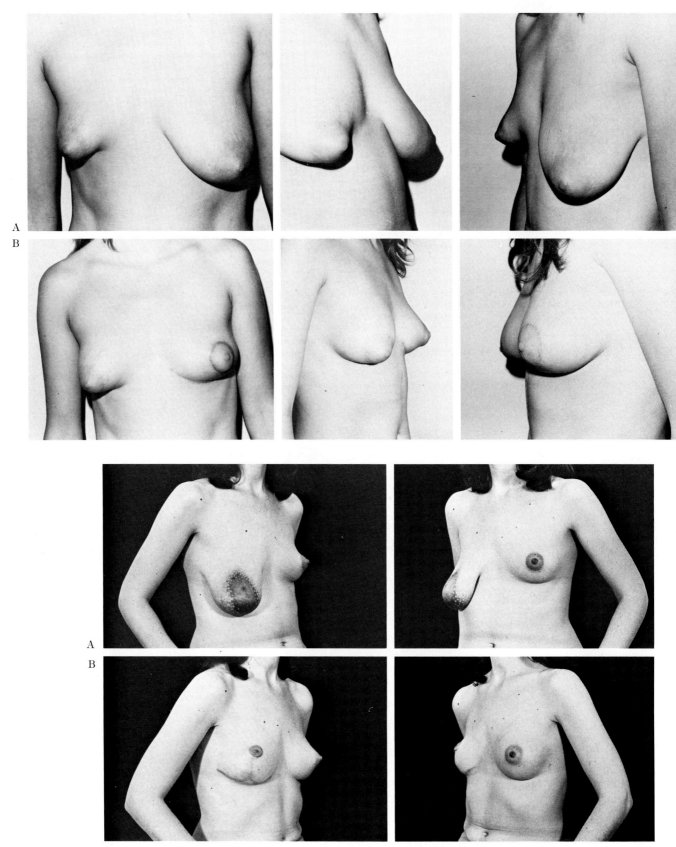

◀ **FIG. 4–10.**
The most difficult asymmetric condition to correct is a combination of hyper- and hypomastia **(A).** In spite of a carefully planned augmentation on one side and reduction on the other **(B),** the symmetry is less than ideal.

◀ **FIG. 4–11.**
A combination of severe ptosis and mild hypomastia **(A),** requiring correction by elevation of one side and augmentation of the other **(B).** (See Operative Sequence IV in this chapter.)

augmentation on one side and a reduction on the other is the simplest solution. Like most simple solutions, however, the end result is often suboptimal (Fig. 4-10A, B).

The hypoplastic breast, in addition to its lack of bulk, is frequently ptotic. In this situation, a mammapexy, with or without simultaneous augmentation, will be necessary. This should almost always be performed **before** reducing the contralateral breast, because a reduction is a more flexible procedure. Varying the degree of resection may be necessary to match the side which has more fixed landmarks. However, in the following case (shown pre- and postoperatively in Fig. 4-11) the reverse sequence was used. In this situation the hypertrophy was associated with quite marked ptosis, and it was felt wiser to reduce and lift the hypertrophic breast to the greatest extent possible. The hypoplastic side was then augmented with an inflatable prosthesis to match the operated side.

A conventional keyhole pattern was marked (in the upright position) on the ptotic breast, elevating the future nipple site to match the other side (IV-1).

IV-1

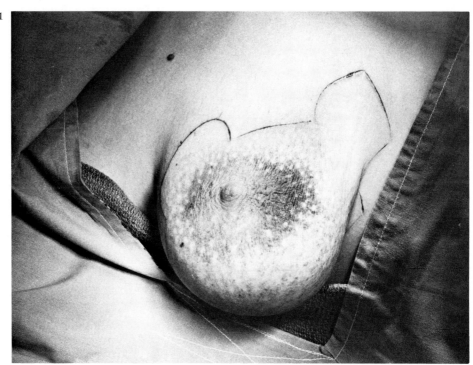

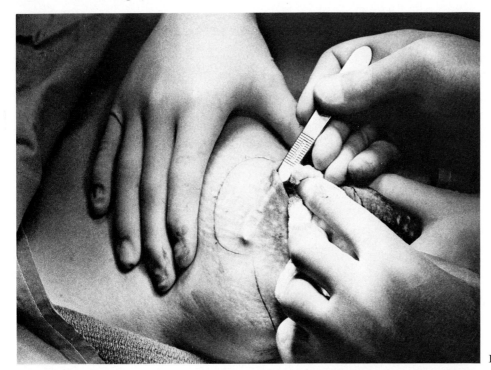

IV-2

IV-3

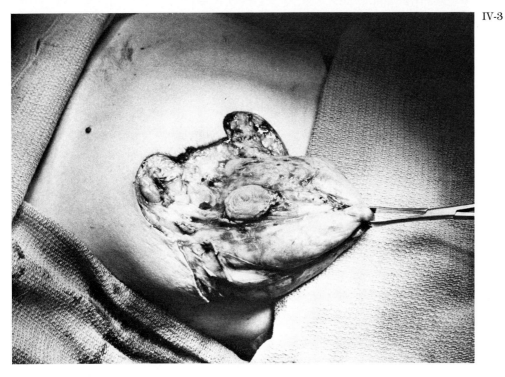

The nipple was reduced to a diameter of 5 cm., and the adjacent skin de-epithelialized (IV-2). The excess skin was resected (IV-3), and the ptotic breast tissue plicated into a "bundle" (IV-4). The viable nipple was elevated into its destination (IV-5) and a taut closure achieved over drains (IV-6).

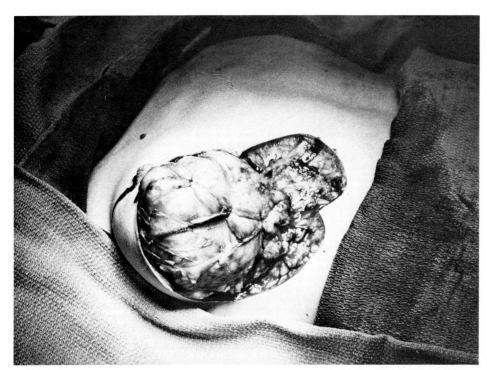

IV-4

IV-5

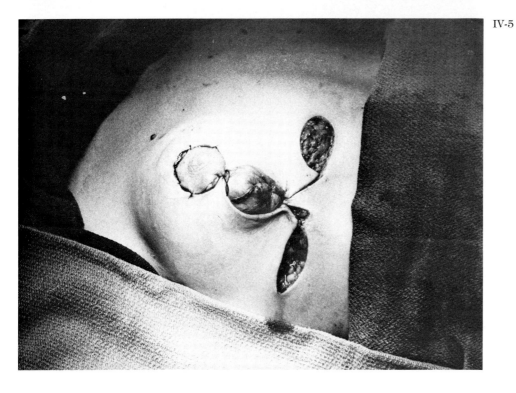

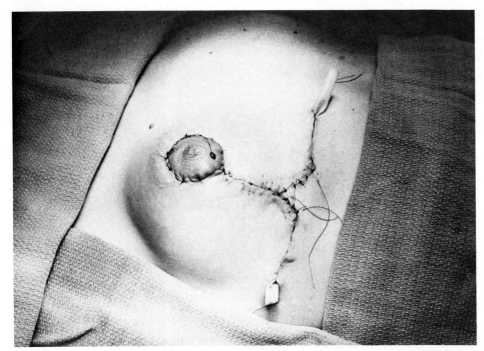

IV-6

IV-7

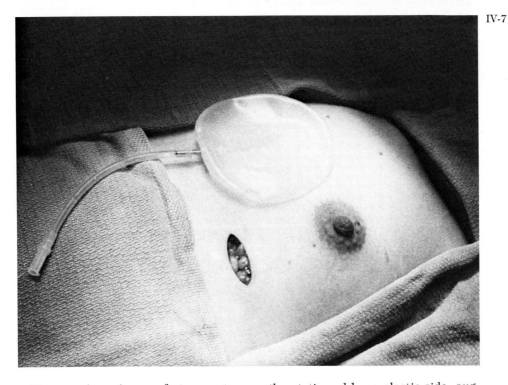

Having achieved a satisfactory contour on the ptotic and hyperplastic side, augmentation of the opposite breast was begun. A small (1-inch) incision was made in the inframammary fold, and with sharp and blunt dissection a pocket was dissected behind the breast (IV-7). An inflatable implant was inserted (IV-8) and filled until a good "match" was achieved (IV-9).

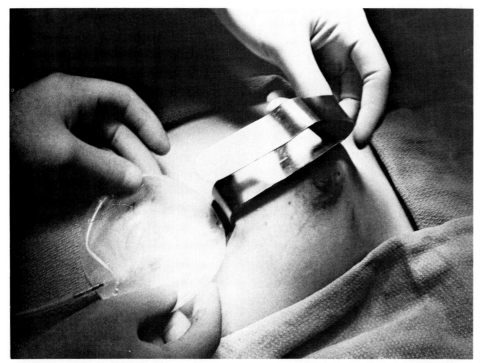

IV-8

IV-9

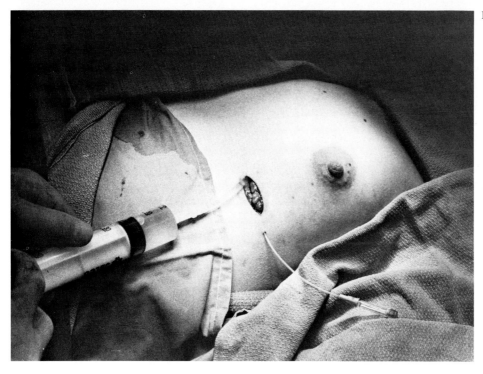

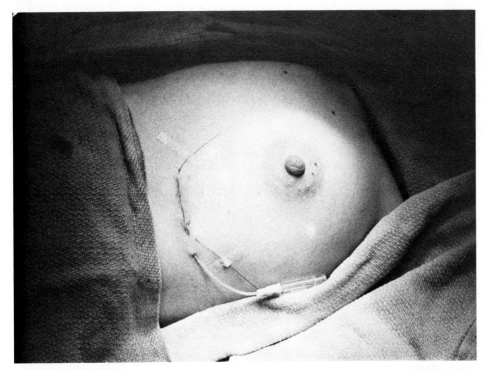

IV-10

IV-11

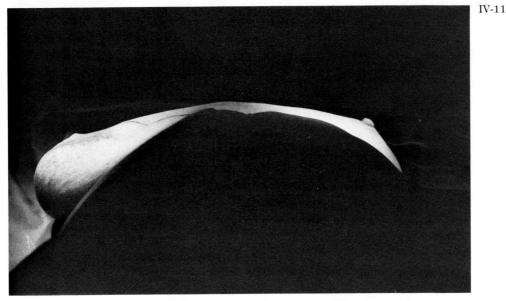

Closure was conventional over an Intracath left indwelling for subsequent instillation of triamcinolone (IV-10).

The sequence of events is well demonstrated by the photographs. The preoperative situation in the recumbent position is shown (IV-11). After skin reduction and correction of ptosis, the change of the shape is clearly shown (IV-12). Finally, the opposite breast is shown inflated to the correct degree (IV-13).

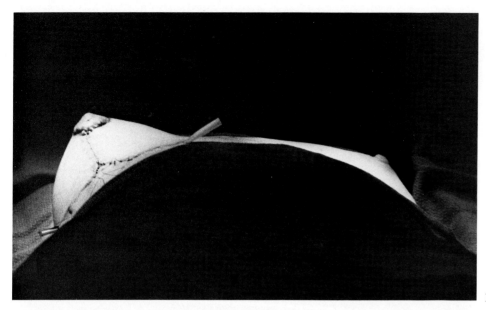

IV-12

IV-13

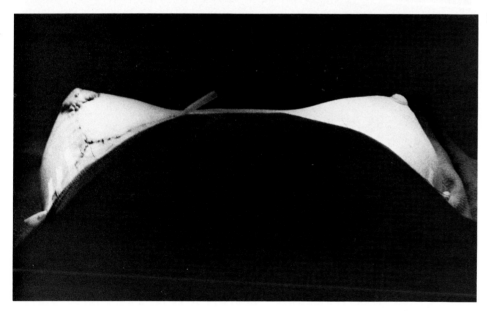

To avoid the cardinal error of producing breasts with nipples of uneven height, it is mandatory to mark both breasts in the upright position and to plan the future position of the nipples before proceeding with the resection of breast skin and the resection or augmentation of bulk.

ASYMMETRIC HYPOMASTIA

In its most straightforward form, this is the easiest asymmetric condition to correct, requiring aug-

mentations of unequal degree. Either gel-filled prostheses of different sizes may be used, or, according to preference, inflatable prostheses may be inserted and filled with saline until the required degree of augmentation is reached.

However, this simple approach is only valid if the nipples are at the same height. If there is a discrepancy in nipple position, this must be corrected by a unilateral or bilateral mammapexy before proceeding with the augmentation (Fig. 4-12A, B).

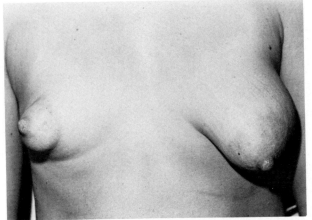

FIG. 4–12.
Asymmetric hypomastia **(A)** treated by elevation of the larger breast and asymmetric augmentation of both **(B).**

A

B

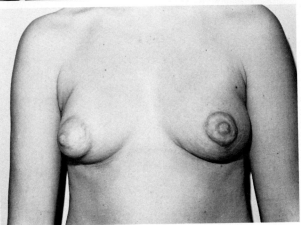

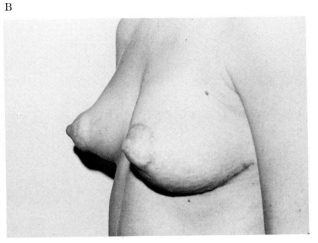

ASYMMETRIC HYPERMASTIA

Correction of this condition is conceptually simple, involving a bilateral asymmetric reduction mammaplasty. Preplanned incisions, with the nipple location at an identical height, are made. Judicious resection of unequal quantities of breast tissue is accomplished to afford postoperative symmetry.

COMPLICATIONS

The complications attendant upon either augmentation or reduction mammaplasty all may follow correction of breast asymmetry. These have been described in detail previously and need not be dealt with here. The less-than-ideal result (and we all have different standards) will usually be a consequence of less-than-ideal planning rather than technical mishaps.

AUTHOR'S CHOICE OF PROCEDURE

As can be seen from the preceding descriptions, there are no "magic solutions" to the correction of breast asymmetry, and the author certainly has no original operative procedures to present. I would, however, make a plea that a most careful assessment of the abnormality be performed, in terms of which procedure, or combination of procedures, will yield the truly optimal result.

This assessment is difficult when judging the disparity of bulk by eye alone, although the experienced surgeon can usually achieve acceptable results. It is useful in planning the extent of breast resection, or, for that matter, the degree of necessary augmentation, to have an accurate measurement of the volume, or displacement, of each breast recorded prior to starting the procedure. Several devices have been described to accomplish this quantitative assessment; the simplest

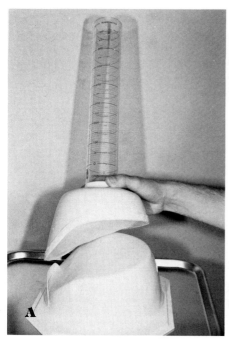
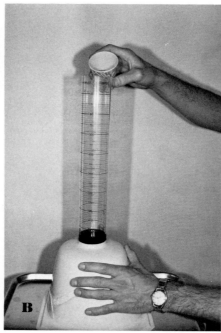
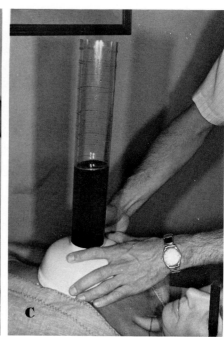

FIG. 4–13.
A. The Tegtmeier mammometer, showing the graduated cylinder, the flexible diaphragm, and the thorax-shaped base. **B.** Filling the mammometer on its base to the zero mark. **C.** Measuring the volume displacement of a breast.

and most reliable is the mammometer devised by Tegtmeier and manufactured by Cosmetech (Fig. 4-13A, B, C).

As plastic surgeons we must all be perfectionists; where an easy operation will produce a less-than-ideal result, surely we should have the imagination to devise a procedure, possibly only applicable to one patient every ten years, to yield the best possible result for that patient.

REFERENCES

1. **Dufourmentel C, Mouly R:** Plastie mammire par la méthode oblique. Ann Chir Plast 6:1, 1961
2. **Elliot RA Jr, Hoehn JG:** Asymmetrical breasts. In Georgrade NG (ed): Reconstructive Breast Surgery. St Louis, Mosby, 1976
3. **McKissock PK:** Reduction mammaplasty: the vertical dermal flap. Plas Reconstr Surg 49:245, 1972
4. **Olivari N:** The latissimus flap. Br J Plast Surg 29:126, 1976
5. **Penn J:** Breast reduction. Br J Plast Surg 7:357, 1955
6. **Strombeck JO:** Mammaplasty: report of a new technique based on the two-pedicle procedure. Br J Plast Surg 13:79, 1960
7. **Trier WC:** Complete breast absence. Plast Reconstr Surg 36:430, 1965

5

treatment of chronic fibrocystic disease

Although the incidence of fibrocystic disease of the breast is not known with certainty, it is a very common condition among women, particularly those who are in their 30s or older. It is postulated that, at some time in their lives, over 50 per cent of women are afflicted with this condition. It is characterized by recurrent nodularity of the breasts, in many cases associated with pain, particularly at the time of the menstrual period.

The pathology of fibrocystic disease may take different forms.[5] They include:

1. Simple cysts and dilated ducts
2. Sclerosing and florid adenosis
3. Fibrosis of the breast stroma
4. Duct epithelial hyperplasia
5. Apocrine metaplasia

Any of these major components of the disease may be present in varying proportions.

Chronic fibrocystic disease per se is a benign entity, although there is a suggestion that the last two histologic patterns, duct epithelial hyperplasia and apocrine metaplasia, may represent a higher risk of pre-malignancy than the other features. The cellular appearance of these is shown in Figure 5-1A and B. However, the appearance of any masses within the glandular substance of the breast demands diagnostic maneuvers, either aspiration or a formal biopsy. With the increasing sophistication of radiographic techniques (mammography, xeroradiography, and now the CAT scanner), the necessity for biopsy has been lessened. These techniques are, however, not 100 per cent reliable, and only a brave or foolish surgeon (or patient) allows the presence of a mass in the breast to go undiagnosed.

Thus, chronic fibrocystic disease is an entity which requires continual biopsies of recurrent nodularities to rule out carcinoma. The question of whether chronic fibrocystic disease is an actual precursor of breast cancer is, as yet, uncertain. Numerous authors are convinced that there is an increased incidence of breast carcinoma in patients suffering from fibrocystic disease[5] particularly when there is a high family incidence of carcinoma.

All studies suggesting a direct cause-and-effect relationship are retrospective and hence somewhat suspect.

In the judgment of this author, the controversy is moot. Recurrent nodularity of the breast, particularly when associated with disabling pain, is, as will be detailed later, an indication for resection of the glandular portion of the breast, regardless of whether or not fibrocystic disease is felt to be a precursor of breast cancer.

HISTORIC ASPECTS

Until the past 10 or 15 years, there were only two courses of treatment available to the patient suffering, as described, from chronic fibrocystic disease.

The first, and more radical, approach was the performance of a simple mastectomy, which entailed the removal of the glandular portion of the breasts together with some overlying skin, including the nipple. This procedure left the patient with an entirely defeminized chest contour with long scars replacing the nipples. Obviously, an external prosthesis had to be worn to restore some degree of symmetry when the patient was clothed; the patient's choice of clothing would be very limited by the scarring and deformity imposed by the operation. This somewhat drastic approach would properly be reserved for the most serious of cases.

The second approach available was a very conservative one, consisting of observation of the breasts, with biopsies being performed as masses recurred. This conservative philosophy imposed tremendous emotional strain on the patient, who would repeatedly present herself for a breast biopsy never knowing whether or not she would awaken from anesthesia to find that a radical mastectomy had been performed for cancer. In addition, the biopsy of discrete masses does little to relieve the often severe mastodynia, a common associated symptom of chronic fibrocystic disease.

With the advent of breast implant technology, it became apparent that a middle course between these two extremes was possible. Freeman[3] pion-

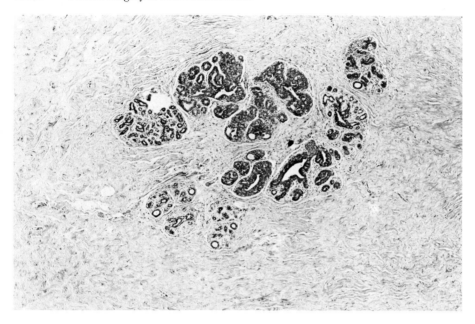

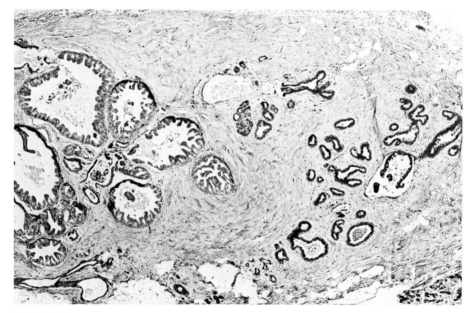

FIG. 5–1.
A. Duct epithelial hyperplasia. B. Apocrine metaplasia.

eered the concept of resection of the diseased glandular tissue of the breast, followed by replacement with a silastic-gel prosthesis. Thus, both aims of surgery could be achieved: on the one hand, removal of the diseased breast tissue, and on the other hand, replacement of the resected bulk to restore some semblance of femininity to the chest contour. This basic concept has undergone some modification since first described but in essence remains the procedure of choice for chronic fibrocystic disease when surgery is indicated (see Author's Choice).

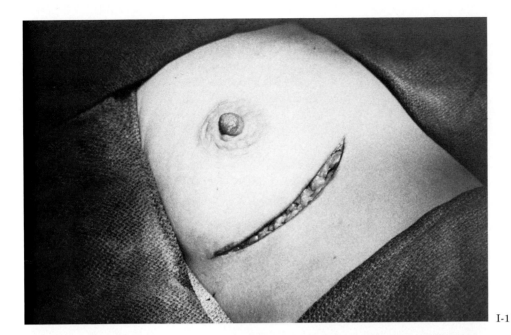

I-1

I-2

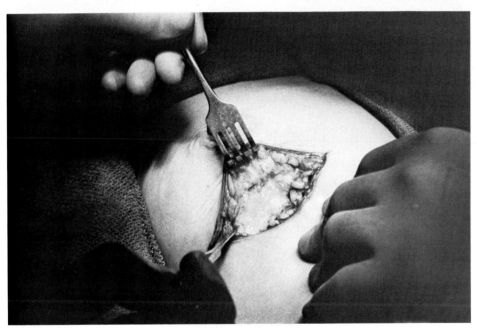

CONTEMPORARY PROCEDURES

TECHNIQUE

Single-Stage Resection and Reconstruction

Resection of the glandular portion of the breast may be carried out either with an inframammary incision (I-1) (longer than that used for augmentation mammaplasty) or a breast-splitting operation consisting of a horizontal excision across the meridian of the breast curving around the inferior portion of the areola. The breast tissue is readily exposed through either of these incisions.

Initially, the mammary gland is dissected, with sharp and blunt dissection, from the pectoralis fascia (I-2).

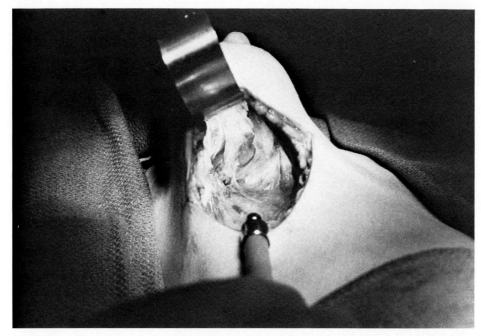

I-3

I-4

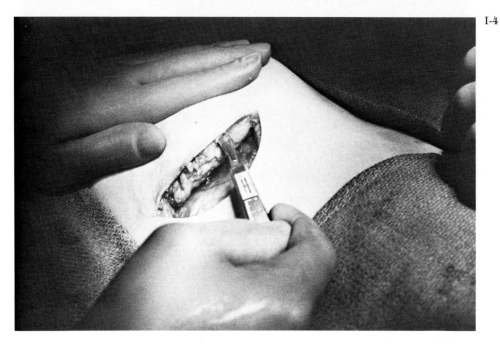

The dissection proceeds to the midline, beyond the lateral margin of the breast, superiorly to the clavicle, and between the humeral and pectoral origins of the pectoralis major muscle to resect as much of the tail of Spence as possible (I-3). The more proximal axillary lymph nodes may be removed to provide further diagnostic material for the pathologist.

The more difficult aspect of the dissection involves the separation of the superior aspect of the gland from the undersurface of the skin with its attached subcutaneous tissue (I-4, I-5, I-6).

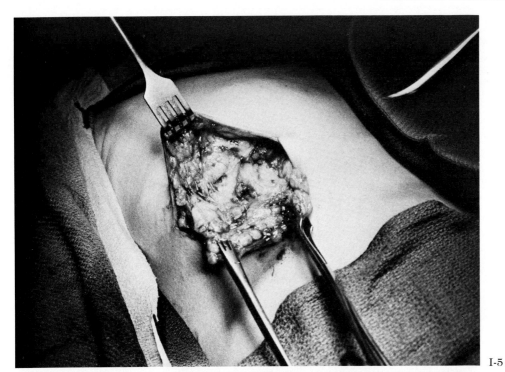

I-5

I-6

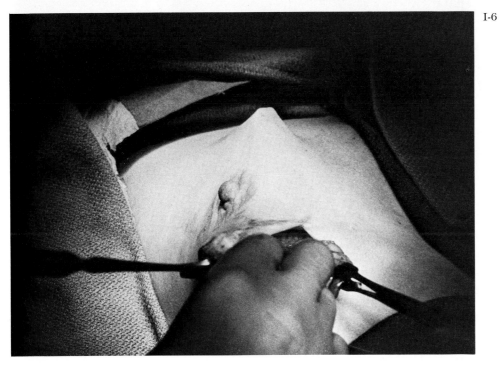

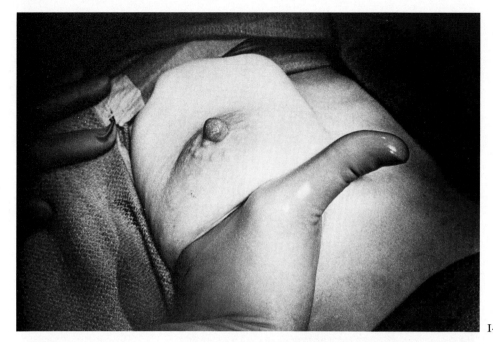

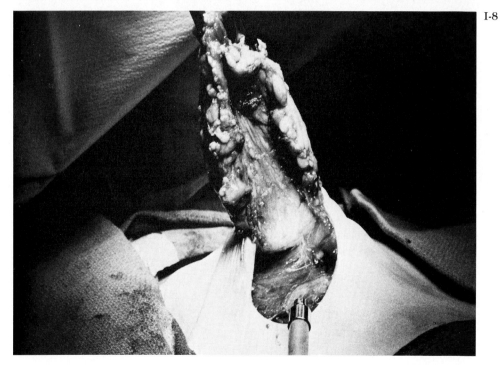

This dissection usually proceeds sharply and must involve the same area as was dissected behind the mammary gland (I-7). The incisions are then connected and the entire breast gland is removed in one portion (I-8, I-9). The dissection is tedious and often bloody, in many cases requiring blood replacement. For this reason it is advised that prior to surgery the patient provide two units of blood for autotransfusion, just as with a reduction mammaplasty.

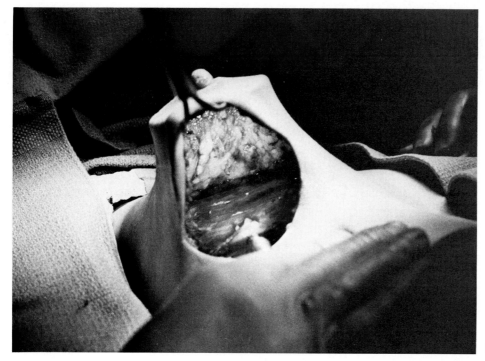

I-9

It must also be recognized that only from 90 to 95 per cent of all breast tissue is removed during this procedure.[4] Not only will some breast tissue be left below the areola, but even though a conscientious attempt is made to remove all breast tissue from the skin flaps (and the resection should **never** be jeopardized by leaving breast tissue for the sake of thicker and more secure skin flaps), small but significant quantities of breast tissue are left, and may remain, in the axilla, the epigastrium, and further distant portions of the thorax. The resected specimen is sent to the pathology department, where very detailed examination is performed to determine whether there is occult breast carcinoma (6 to 10% occurring in Pennisi's series[5]).

The reconstruction of a breast which has undergone subcutaneous mastectomy has evolved through many modifications since Freeman's original description of a one-stage subcutaneous replacement. We ourselves have followed the evolution of this reconstruction carefully, and have in general paralleled the national trend. Initially, reconstruction was accomplished by means of an immediate replacement of the resected gland by a silastic implant in the orthotopic position (i.e., placed subcutaneously).

This procedure was by and large satisfactory (Fig. 5-2A, B); however, many serious complications of skin slough, with exposure of the implant necessitating removal, were reported[1]. In addition, the rather thick-walled seamed implant available at that time (the 1960s) was quite readily palpable, and on some occasions visible, beneath the rather thin skin, because it was unprotected by the interposition of normal breast tissue for its camouflage (Fig. 5-3A, B). In short, it was felt that a direct subcutaneous replacement was both risky and in many cases aesthetically left a great deal to be desired.

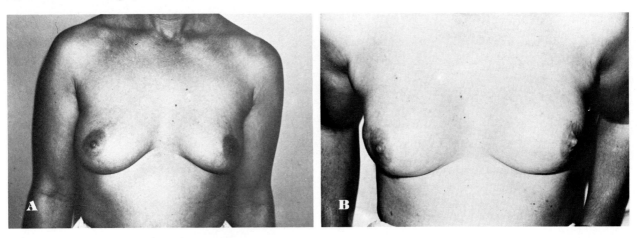

FIG. 5–2.
A. Preoperative fibrocystic disease. B. Following subcutaneous mastectomy with one-stage orthotopic augmentation.

FIG. 5–3.
A. One-stage subcutaneous mastectomy and reconstruction preoperatively. B. Postoperatively, showing capsular contracture with a palpable prosthesis.

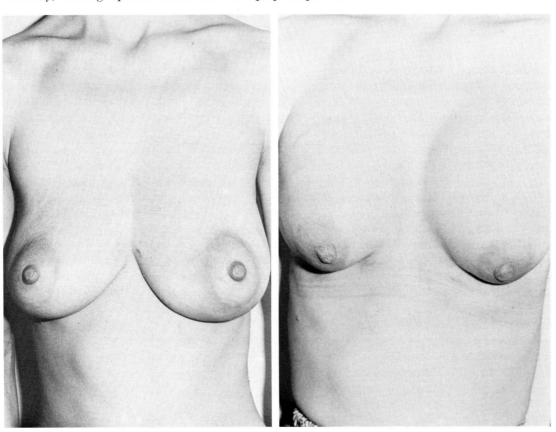

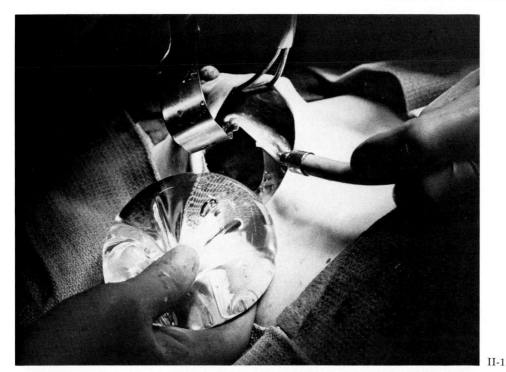

II-1

II-2

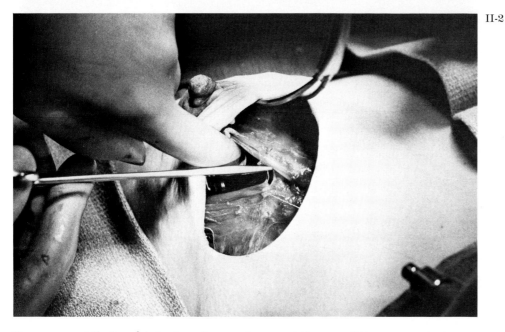

Dempsey and Latham[2] introduced a novel concept for permitting a one-stage procedure without risking the survival of skin flaps. Following the resection, this involved developing a new plane between the rib cage and the pectoralis major muscle and insertion of the implant in a subpectoral location (II-1). Not only did this allow bruised skin flaps to heal by virtue of their proximity to the pectoral muscle without the interposition of an impermeable prosthesis, but also the outlines of the implant were blurred by means of its positioning beneath the pectoral muscle (II-2, II-3).

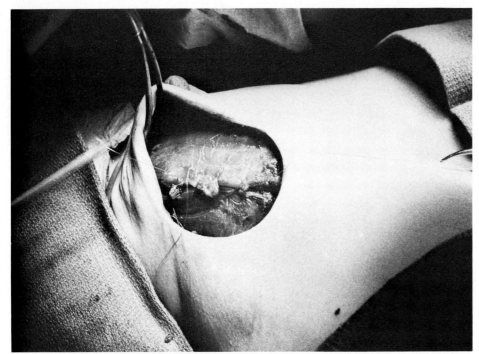

II-3

II-4

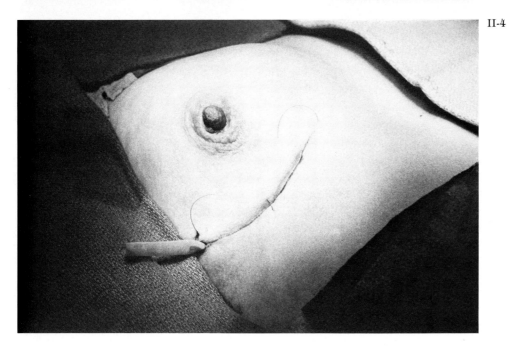

In repose, this procedure offered a more normal-appearing breast (II-4); however, when the pectoral muscles contracted, they could be seen to "cut in" to the prosthesis. Occasionally this procedure has been followed by greater long-range discomfort than reconstruction in the orthotopic position. The pre- and postoperative status of the patient undergoing the single-stage procedure described is portrayed in II-5, II-6, II-7, and II-8.

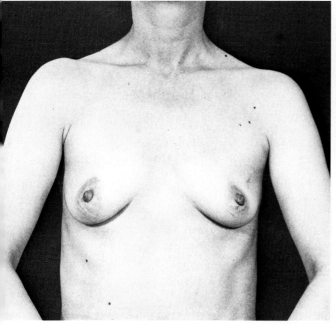
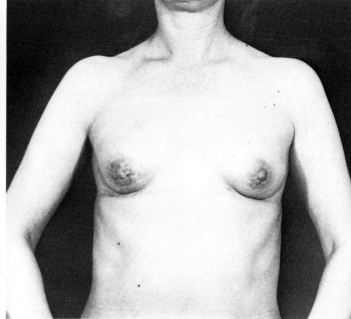

II-5

II-7

II-6

II-8

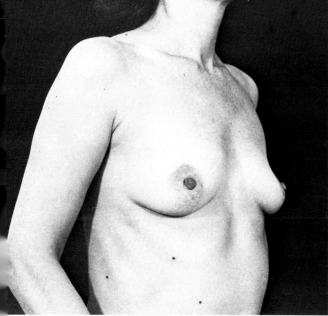
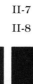
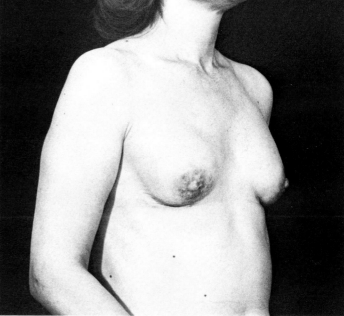

Two-Stage Resection and Reconstruction

Following resection of the entire breast (as already described), the remaining thin skin flaps may show evidence of impaired vascularity. In this situation, a two-stage procedure must be performed. The resection is completed and the wounds closed over a drain. The injured skin flaps are allowed to heal, thicken up, and develop a better vascularity. When the situation appears propitious, a second-stage replacement is performed, in our hands delaying the reconstruction for from three to six months (Fig. 5-4A, B, C).

The drawbacks to this staged procedure were twofold:

1. The patient was forced to undergo a period of relative mutilation to which was added the expense and morbidity of two hospital procedures.

2. As the skin flaps retracted (and this was a considerable problem in the larger ptotic breasts), healing could be most irregular, resulting in a furrowed and unattractive breast skin (Fig. 5-5).

This, in general, was not relieved by the internal stretching afforded by the replacement prosthesis.

Improved Implants

The most recent development in breast reconstruction has been in prosthesis technology; the newer implants are both softer than the older models used in the previous decade and also seamless rather than having a palpable edge. Therefore, an implant can be placed subcutaneously without its appearance being very noticeable, thus precluding the necessity to place this implant under the pectoral muscle for an aesthetic optimum. However, this has made no difference in the selec-

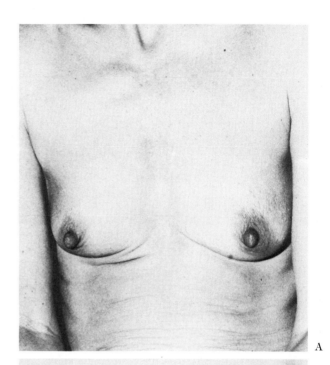

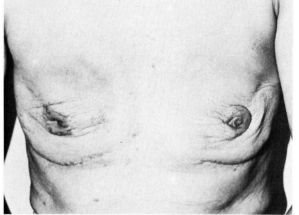

A

B

C

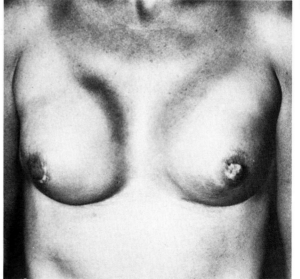

FIG. 5-4.
A. Two-stage subcutaneous mastectomy, with delayed reconstruction, preoperatively. B. Following mastectomy. C. Following reconstruction three months later.

tion of operation where the circulation to the skin overlying the breasts has been impaired by a necessarily thin dissection of the skin flaps.

The choice of operation, then, still depends on an accurate assessment of the condition of the circulation in the skin; when this is so marginal that it will not tolerate the additional insult of being stretched, a two-stage procedure must be employed.

Limitations of Reconstruction

The uncertain nature of the reconstruction **must** be explained to the patient prior to surgery. No guaranty can be made that the operation can be performed in one stage. It must also be very straightforwardly explained to the patient that this is not a cosmetic procedure and most emphatically that it will not produce a normal-appearing breast. There is always some degree, however slight, of deformity resulting from this operation.

A few cases end up with a totally unsatisfactory-appearing breast which the patient may prefer to have removed. It is quite important, in this day of legal responsibility for informed consent, to explain this fortunately rare situation to the patient so that she can make up her own mind as to whether the aesthetic hazards justify the operation.

FIG. 5-5.

The marked skin contracture which can follow subcutaneous mastectomy.

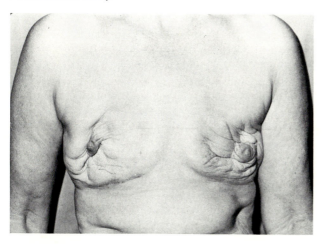

SPECIAL SITUATIONS

Fibrocystic Disease Associated With Ptosis

An additional operative problem is imposed when the breast is large, ptotic, and pendulous. When the breast tissue is resected, a large, empty skin sack is left "flopping" on the chest wall. Whether or not an immediate reconstruction is technically feasible, the excess skin and low nipple position will present a major difficulty in obtaining as good an aesthetic result as possible.

Excess skin must be trimmed so that the skin envelope is appropriate for the size, not of its previous contents, but of the prosthesis employed for its replacement. If this is not performed, the redundant skin will shrink in a totally unpredictable, often asymmetric and generally unacceptable manner, yielding an end result that is unhappy for all parties concerned.

This skin reduction may be accomplished in either of two ways, depending on the degree of ptosis.

Minor Ptosis

When the ptosis and consequent skin excess is relatively minor, the entire operation is planned differently than previously described. A keyhole pattern, positioned so as to elevate the nipples appropriately, is used to outline the area of skin to be resected (Fig. 5-6A).

The nipple is circumscribed intradermally and preserved on a superiorly based dermal pedicle. The excess skin is resected as outlined, and excellent exposure is afforded to the breast, which is then removed as completely as possible. (Fig. 5-6B).

The nipple is brought into position to the superior part of the keyhole by folding, as loosely as possible, its dermal pedicle (Fig. 5-6C). The decision is then made, on the basis of the vascularity and perceived viability of the skin flaps, whether or not to complete the reconstruction in a single stage. If the skin and, importantly, the nipple appear pink and viable, an implant of carefully chosen size may be inserted either orthotopically (Fig. 5-6D) or beneath the pectoral muscle, and the skin flaps are closed conventionally (Fig. 5-6E).

If there is the least hint of cyanosis of the skin, or if capillary refill is retarded to any significant degree, the reconstruction is delayed until the circu-

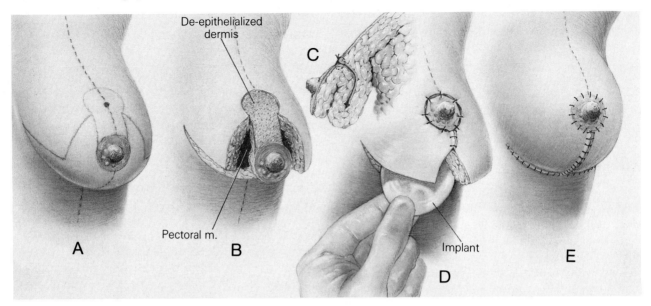

De-epithelialized dermis

C

Pectoral m.

A   B

Implant

D

E

FIG. 5–6.

Correction of minor ptosis associated with fibrocystic disease. A. The keyhole pattern with an outlined superiorly based dermal flap. B. The mastectomy completed, with the nipple surviving on the short dermal flap. C. The nipple is elevated into position by folding the dermal flap. D. An implant of appropriate size is inserted. E. Skin closure is completed.

lation to the skin seems to have recovered from its surgical insult. As a matter of routine, many cautious surgeons prefer to carry out the procedure in two stages to minimize the risk of vascular compromise of the skin.

Major Ptosis

If the degree of ptosis is major, or if the breasts are significantly large and pendulous, the dermal pedicle for the nipple, if fashioned as just described, will be too long and attenuated to support the blood supply (Fig. 5-7A). In such cases a totally different approach will be necessary, involving breast amputation with preservation and "banking" of the nipples in another location, usually the lower abdomen, for storage and subsequent reimplantation.

This, of course, necessitates a two-stage operation. At the first operation, skin flaps are planned similar to those already described and the excess skin is removed. Prior to this, the nipples are reduced in diameter and taken off as free composite grafts. Two equivalent circles of epidermis are removed from any appropriate location, and the nipples are sewn down as free grafts (Fig. 5-7B). The operation then proceeds with resection of redundant skin and all of the breast tissue. The skin flaps are closed and the area left to settle down for several months.

At the time of reconstruction, an inframammary incision is opened and, without dissecting the skin from the pectoral muscle, a plane is developed between the under side of the pectoral muscle and the rib cage. The implant is then inserted behind the pectoral muscle and a disk of epidermis is removed from the apex of each breast. The "banked" nipples are then reimplanted into their correct position, and the donor deficit is closed appropriately (Fig. 5-7C). This two-staged procedure is safe and has been uniformly successful in our hands where needed.

An alternative approach to the "giant" breast is illustrated in the following unusual case, planned with great ingenuity by my colleague, Dr. A. W. Mayer, Jr., in 1966.

A 14-year-old child presented with rapidly enlarging breasts entirely occupied by firm masses, many of which were the size of a tennis ball. At the time of examination the breasts were already massive (Fig. 5-8A), and the emotional disturbance re-

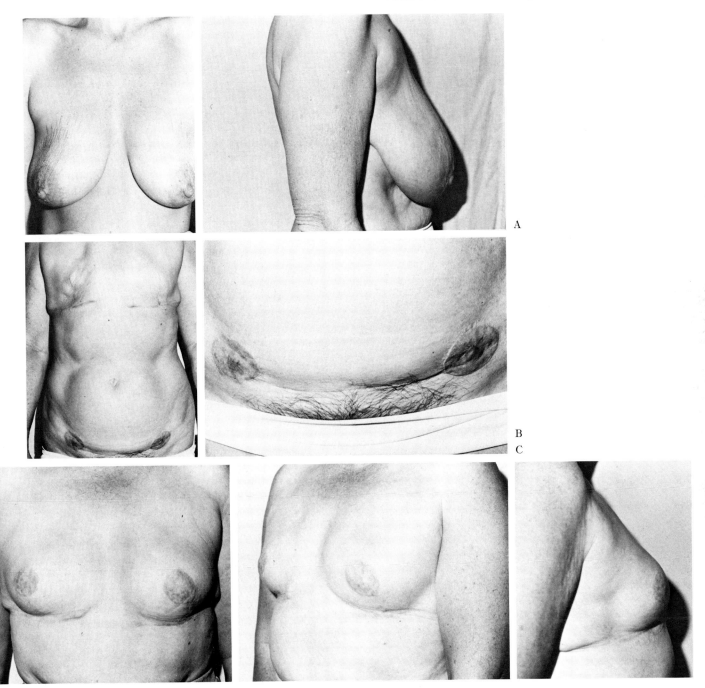

FIG. 5–7.

A. Fibrocystic disease associated with moderately severe ptosis. B. Following subcutaneous mastectomy, reduction of skin, and banking of the nipples in the groin. C. After reconstruction with subpectoral implants and regrafting of the nipples.

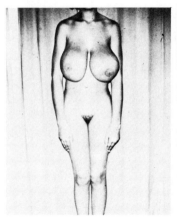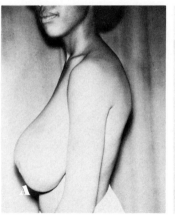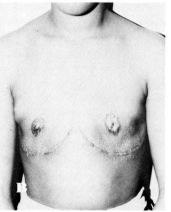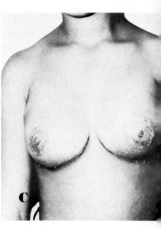

FIG. 5–8.
A. An adolescent with massive breast hypertrophy and multiple fibroadenomas. B. Following subcutaneous mastectomy, skin resection, and free-grafting of the nipples. C. Delayed reconstruction with breast prostheses.

sulting from the deformity was so severe as to require hospitalization.

After a preliminary biopsy showed multiple fibroadenomas, a two-stage procedure was executed. The first stage involved a resection of redundant skin and all of the diseased breast tissue, using a modified Thorek approach. At the same time, the nipples were reduced in size and transplanted as free grafts to the proper location on the anterior skin flap. The nipples took well and healed without loss of bulk (Fig. 5-8B).

At the second stage, four months later, the inframammary incision was reopened and a "medium" Cronin implant was inserted subcutaneously (Fig. 5-8C). There were no complications, and the patient, with no further emotional problems, finished high school to become a very competent nurse.

Silicone Injections

A further indication for subcutaneous mastectomy followed by reconstruction is when liquid silicone has been injected into the breast, producing either nodularity of the breast tissue or skin changes such as discoloration or silicone plaque formation. The operation is necessary in this circumstance because the nodularity of siliconoma formation is impossible to distinguish from neoplasia.

The operation will be more difficult than a "normal" subcutaneous mastectomy because the silicone will have infiltrated the tissues and the skin, making the dissection harder.

In many cases, the silicone will be adherent to the undersurface of the dermis and must be scraped off that structure without, hopefully, endangering the blood supply. In the author's experience, several cases of this type have been followed by skin necrosis, requiring in, some cases, flaps from a distant source for reconstruction (see Chap. 2, Fig. 2-6).

COMPLICATIONS

Statistically, the most common complication is that of skin necrosis overlying a directly implanted prosthesis, with consequent exposure of the implant necessitating its removal. Skin necrosis usually occurs in the lower lateral quadrant of the breast where the circulation to the skin is the poorest. Obviously, this complication results from attempting to reconstruct primarily a resected breast in which the circulation is jeopardized. This may be a very subtle decision and it is easy to make this mistake in the worthy desire to subject the patient to only one operation rather than two.

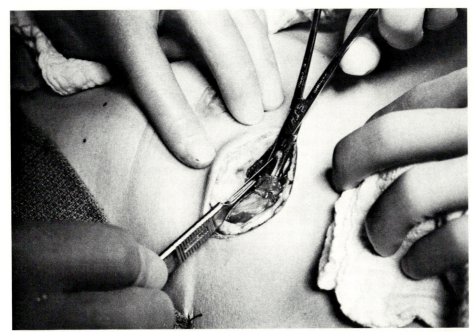

III-1

III-2

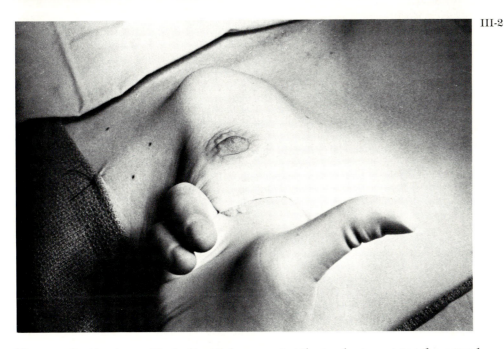

The complication is readily dealt with by removing the implant, excising the ragged edges of skin, and suturing them primarily to create a closed incision. After a delay of a number of weeks to allow for healing and maturation of the scar, the inframammary incision is reopened and the implant replaced (III-1 through III-6). A greater margin of safety would be afforded in this situation by replacing the implant in a subpectoral location to give greater protection to the area of skin which had previously broken down. While this may produce some degree of asymmetry, it is regarded as a safer procedure.

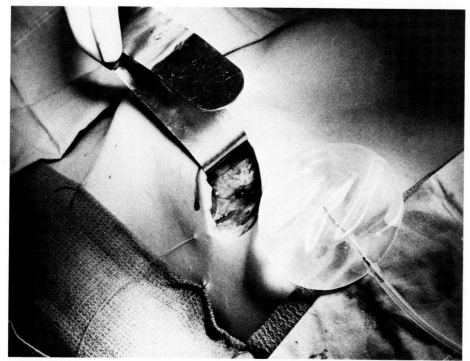

III-3

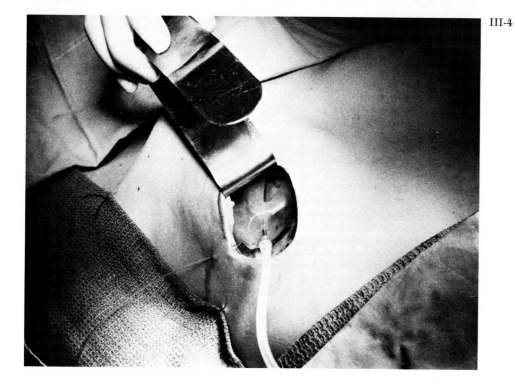

III-4

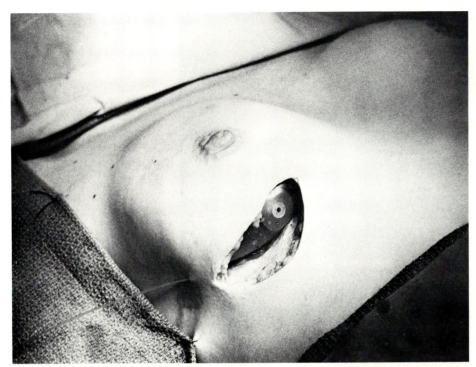

III-5

III-6

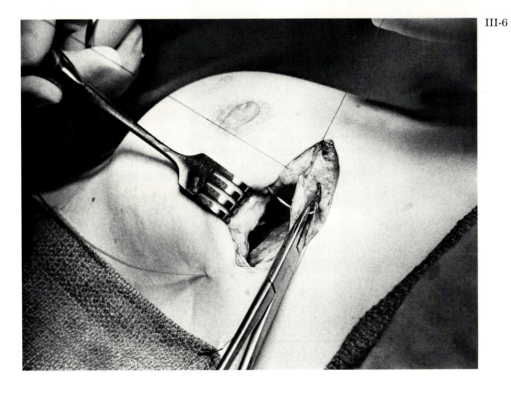

6

reconstruction of the breast following radical mastectomy

WITH DAVID M. CHARLES
AND RICHARD H. McSHANE

There is no question that one of the most exciting frontiers in plastic surgery today is the development of the concept of reconstructing a breast following radical mastectomy. This idea would have been almost unthinkable as recently as 20 years ago, when it was regarded as sacrilege to interfere with the locally healed radical mastectomy scar. It was felt that this would invite earlier recurrence of the disease and adversely affect the survival rate. The very rare patients accepted for reconstruction were limited to those who had initially had a stage-one carcinoma without axillary metastasis and who had additionally survived at least five years.

What has happened in the interim to change the thinking of progressive surgeons specializing in this field?

1. There has been a greater understanding of the biology and natural history of breast carcinoma.[21] It is now recognized that the **local** recurrence rate is small—approximately 10 per cent. Most of these cases occur in advanced tumors with skin fixation at the time of resection.

2. There has been a marked trend away from the "supraradical" procedures, and a progressive disillusionment with the classic Halsted operation, involving a long vertical incision, thin skin flaps, and occasionally application of a split-thickness graft to achieve closure when a wide skin resection had been performed. The "modified radical mastectomy" of Patey[18] with a horizontal incision and sparing of the pectoral musculature, is now generally preferred.

3. Improvement of implant technology and the greater familiarity with the use of silastic prostheses have broadened the acceptance of this procedure.

4. There is much greater understanding of the psychological stress imposed by radical mastectomy with its inevitable loss of the outward symbol of femininity. It is recognized that the desire on the part of the patient to restore her feminine contour is serious and not trivial, and that the aims of reconstructive surgery (i.e., restoration of some degree of symmetry) can be achieved without too much difficulty.

Even though convinced of the benefits of restoration as early as possible of a breast "symbol," we must defer to our general surgery colleagues who have the primary responsibility for the patient both in selection of candidates and choosing the appropriate delay (if any) between resection and reconstruction. It would be completely irresponsible for the plastic surgeon to proceed with a breast reconstruction without having first ascertained the size and location of the resected tumor, its histologic type and degree of invasiveness, and the presence or absence of positive axillary nodes. It would also be a breach of good manners not to discuss the patient's wish for reconstruction with the original surgeon if he has not in fact referred the case, and if possible to obtain his complete assent.

HISTORIC ASPECTS

Since breast reconstruction following radical mastectomy is quite recent, there literally is no historical background to this procedure. The earliest pioneers in the field are still actively describing modifications and improvements to their original procedures.

CONTEMPORARY PROCEDURES

SIMPLE AUGMENTATION

Undoubtedly, the easiest operation to provide a "breast symbol" consists of the placement of an appropriately sized and shaped prosthesis under the healed skin flaps.[20] This procedure may be satisfactory if a "Patey"[18] modified radical mastectomy has been performed, with reasonable laxity of the skin and adequate thick flaps to support the interposition of a prosthesis between the chest musculature and the skin. It has been pointed out by

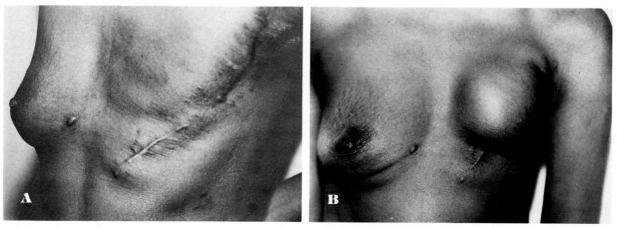

FIG. 6–1.
A. A healed radical mastectomy. B. Reconstruction by simple augmentation.

FIG. 6–2.
Perras' operation, halving a redundant contralateral breast to replace both lost bulk and missing nipple.

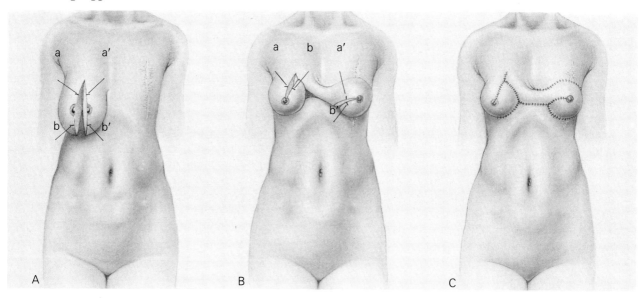

Guthrie[8] that the average patient only requires that she look as normal as possible in a brassiere and clothing without having to resort to an external prosthesis. The results of simple augmentation, however, leave a lot to be desired aesthetically, and they may be technically unsatisfactory when the skin of the breast following resection is tight and scarred (Fig. 6-1A, B).

STAGED FLAP RECONSTRUCTION

Recognizing the disparity in skin area between the normal and operated breast, numerous attempts have been made to provide greater relaxation for the subsequent insertion of a prosthesis. These have involved Perras' use of a pedicle flap from the contralateral breast when this organ is excessively ptotic[19] (Fig. 6-2); abdominal tube pedicles

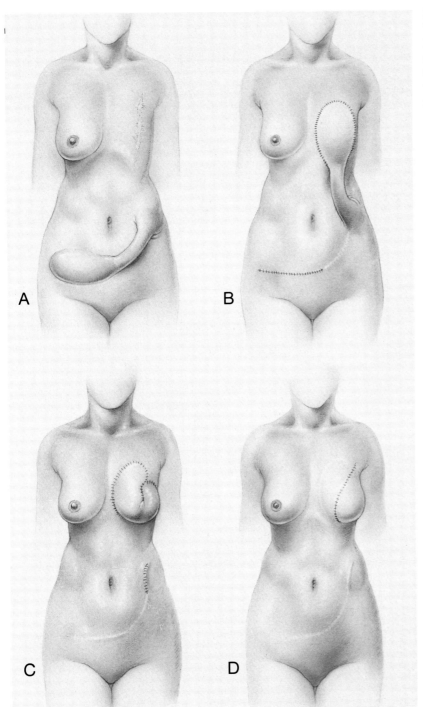

FIG. 6–3.
The Hoehler procedure, which stages a large lower abdominal "paddle" (A), swung into place on a tubed pedicle (B). This pedicle tissue is itself sectioned (C) and incorporated into the reconstruction (D).

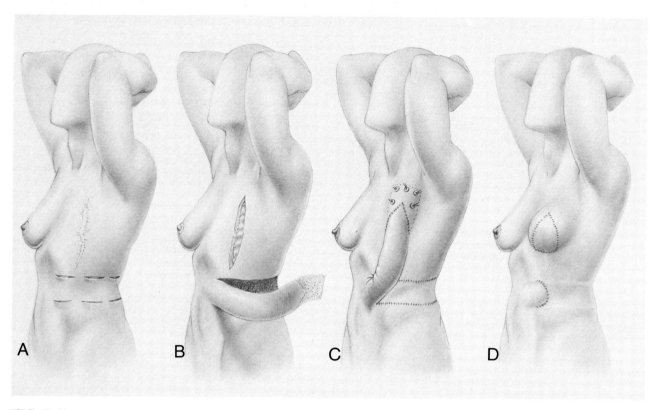

FIG. 6–4.
The Cronin procedure. A long, medially based flap is deflayed, and, with its tip de-epithelialized, swung through 90° to gain relaxation in the vertical axis (A through D).

FIG. 6–5.
The Millard procedure. As with Hoehler's operation, an abdominal tube pedicle is used to augment the tight skin of the chest (A through D).

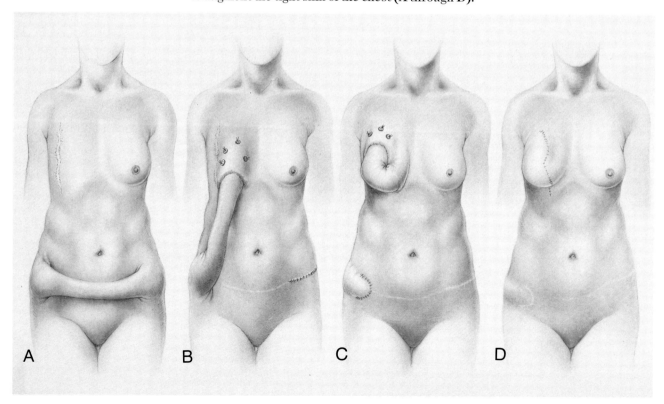

brought up by stages into the location of the breast by Hoehler[9] (Fig. 6-3); and a delayed tube pedicle from the lateral thorax ultimately swung into appropriate position with excellent results by Cronin[5] (Fig. 6-4). Millard (Fig. 6-5), ever the supreme innovator, has also made useful contributions to the field with his variation of the abdominal tube pedicle.[14] A latissimus dorsi flap may also be employed[10] to add bulk and cover. This important procedure will be discussed in greater detail later in this chapter.

These procedures, many of which have been demonstrated to produce superb aesthetic results, pay tribute to the imagination of the pioneering plastic surgeons, both in this country and overseas. Having produced a satisfactory degree of skin and subcutaneous coverage, an implant is inserted to produce as normally bulky a breast as possible. Since it is extremely difficult to mimic a normal structure with a wide range of anatomic variation, it is likely that the contralateral breast will need modification, either by means of augmentation, reduction, or correction of ptosis.

Freeman, a highly experienced surgeon in this field, now recommends a subcutaneous mastectomy followed by reconstruction in the contralateral side, due to the frequency of occult malignant disease in the contralateral breast.[7] Following reconstruction of the breast mound, a nipple may be created either by means of a labial mucosal graft,[1] a graft from the nipple of the contralateral side,[14] or by tattooing pigment to simulate a nipple onto the apex of the reconstructed breast.

To point out the relative newness of the procedure, in the United States in 1977 Cocke and Lynch[4] reported on the results of a questionnaire mailed to all members of the American Society of Plastic and Reconstructive Surgery. Of 800 respondents, only 360 had performed reconstructions following mastectomy for carcinoma. A total of 1200 operations were described, of which about 1000 consisted of the insertion of a mammary prosthesis, and 200 made use of pedicle flap tissue. Overlapping the preceding larger groups, 83 combined the techniques. The surgeons reported an overall satisfactory result in 88 per cent of their cases. There is no doubt that the figures today would be of a considerably greater order of magnitude.

COMPLICATIONS

The principal complication is skin necrosis resulting from a combination of tight, scarred, devascularized skin and flaps which are brought into place under too much tension, thus depriving them of whatever blood supply they may have. If, to this unfavorable situation, we add the additional insult of insertion of an implant, skin necrosis and subsequent exposure of the prosthesis may result. As always, it is a fine point of judgment whether to accept a certain degree of tension or to be extremely cautious and stage the procedure, delaying the insertion of the implant. This will be a matter for the judgment of the individual surgeon who alone can judge the situation best at the operating table, drawing upon his training, skill, and experience in handling tissue with a jeopardized blood supply to make the correct decision. However, flap necrosis and implant exposure requiring removal may occur even with the most skillful and experienced surgeon.

Finally, radiation, quite commonly employed as an adjunct to mastectomy, has significant long-range effects upon tissue and particularly its vascularity. Without dwelling on this complex subject to which many books have been devoted, it can be summed up in three words—"poor wound healing."

The simple insertion of an implant under the cover of radiated skin will generally be self-defeating. Utilizing a pedicle flap which has itself been radiated is similarly foolish; however, when new tissue can be brought from outside the irradiated zone with its own uncompromised blood supply, it will enhance healing in a jeopardized area. Delay, rather than immediate insertion of the implant, is recommended in this instance.

AUTHOR'S CHOICE OF PROCEDURE

Excited by the results obtained by pioneers in the field, and gratified by the acceptance of the concept by general surgeons in our locality, my colleague R. H. McShane and I devised a one-stage reconstruction which would be suitable for almost all cases of healed radical mastectomies. This is in many respects similar to the method developed independently by Bohmert[2] and presented at the Sixth International Congress of Plastic Surgery in 1976.

INDICATIONS

At the present time, we are not performing this procedure as a primary or delayed primary operation, but prefer to let the process of wound healing mature for six months following resection. We are not as radical in our approach as some authors[10] and currently limit reconstruction to those patients who have a lesion of less than 2 cm., no fixation to either skin or deeper structures, and have a maximum of two axillary nodes involved. We feel that this is a reasonable compromise between excessive conservatism and "taking on all comers"; it is quite possible, however, that we may modify our approach and liberalize our indications as more experience is gained both by ourselves and others.

TECHNIQUE

Recognizing that the principal obstacle to a satisfactory contour of a reconstructed breast is the tissue deficiency in the vertical axis overlying the rib cage, we have designed a large Z-plasty which makes use of the laxity in the lateral thoracoabdominal region that most individuals possess. This Z-plasty is quite asymmetric and may be varied in its angulation and the length of the flaps used according to the individual situation. However, the concept, regardless of whether a vertical or horizontal incision has been used, is basically the same and consists of a medially based triangular interpolation flap which is transposed into a vertically planned defect. It can also be utilized where a skin graft has been employed to close the skin defect.

Horizontal Scar

A horizontal incision is employed in the modified radical mastectomy operation described by Patey.[18] The end result of this operation lends itself to reconstruction, and in most instances this has been accomplished by the simple placement of a mammary prosthesis. With the pectoral musculature left relatively undisturbed, there is no "telltale hollow" below the clavicle (often a source of grave discomfort to the patient) and the implant serves to replace the bulk lost by resection of the mammary gland.

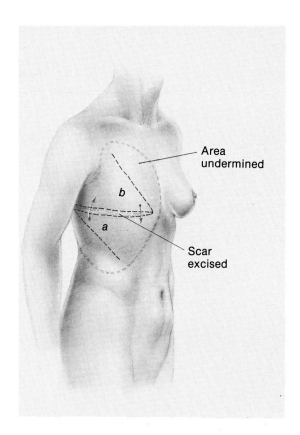

Area
undermined

b

a

Scar
excised

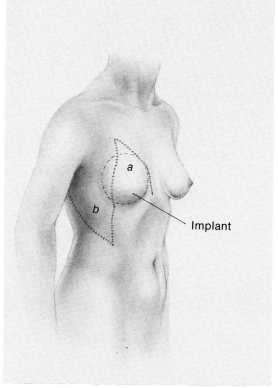

a

b

Implant

I-1

I-2

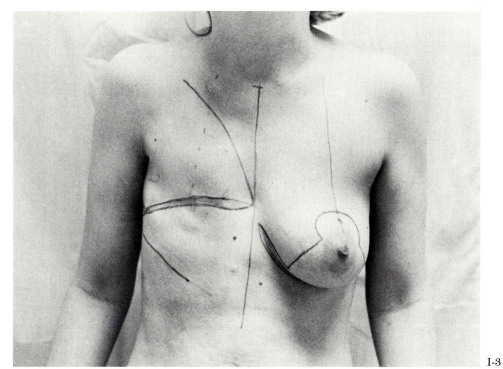

I-3

I-4

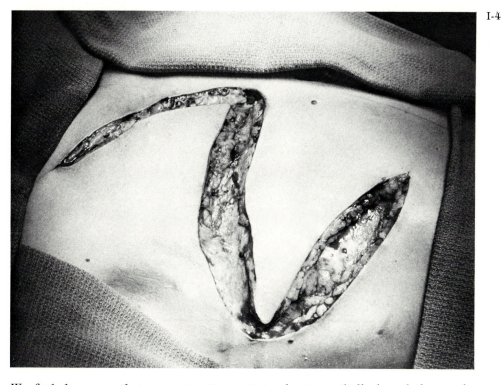

We feel, however, that reconstruction using a large, medially based thoracoab-dominal flap to cover the implant yields an aesthetically more satisfying, as well as a more secure, result (I-1, I-2). The flap is planned as an asymmetric Z-plasty, using the horizontal scar as the central axis of the Z (I-3).

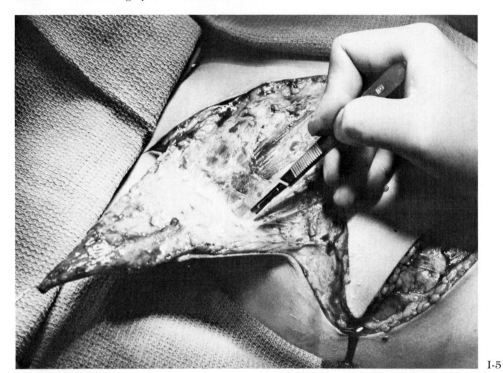

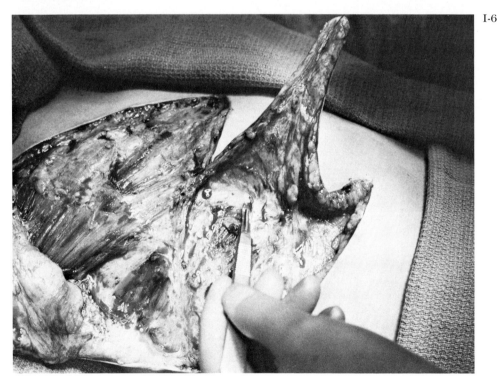

A large triangle, based medially, is swung up into a defect created by an almost vertical incision running from the medial extent of the scar to a point below the clavicle (I-4–I-8).

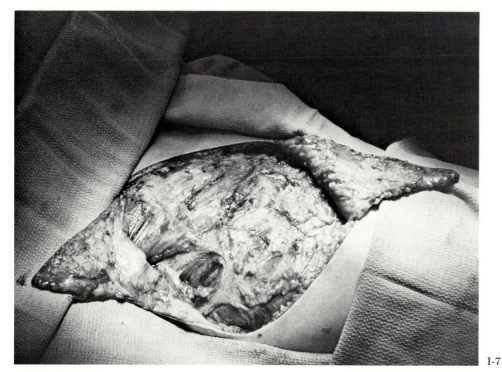

I-7

I-8

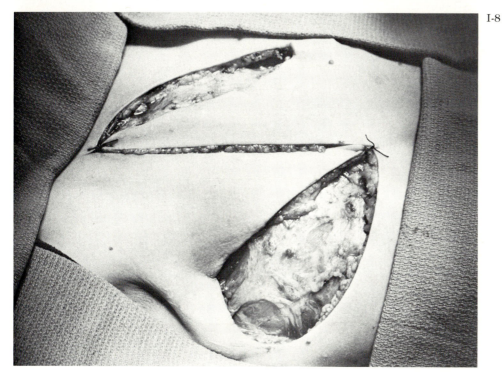

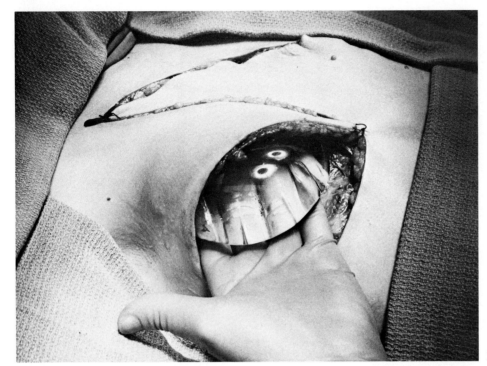

I-9

I-10

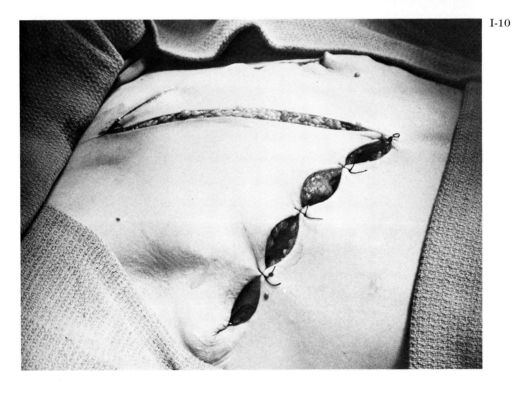

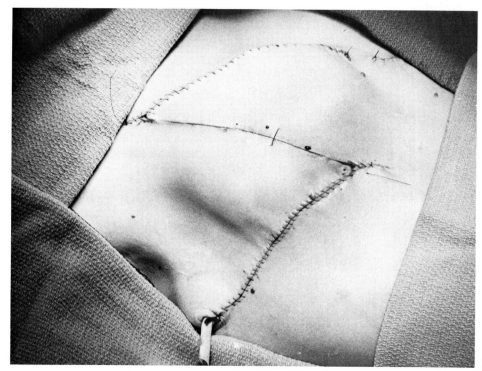

I-11

Undermining is carried out on either side of this vertical incision to allow an adequate pocket for the prosthesis (I-9). Wide undermining is carried out laterally and inferiorly at a level above the external oblique and anterior serratus muscles to allow the flap, which contains the full thickness of the panniculus, to shift vertically and to permit closure of the horizontal defect without undue tension (I-10, I-11).

Although delay of this flap is usually unnecessary due to the fact that the horizontal scar has, in effect, created a delay, a clinical judgment must be made at this point. If the tip of the flap, tacked into position, demonstrates venous engorgement due to the added insult of "kinking" its base, it must be returned to its previous location and subsequent transfer must be delayed for a week to ten days.

This, however, is extremely unusual. A well-designed and adequately mobilized flap will generally survive its transfer with unimpaired vascularity. The laxity thus afforded to the site of previous breast resection will usually permit insertion of a prosthesis of suitable size.

Again, a clinical judgment must be made as to whether to proceed with simultaneous augmentation or to deliberately stage the procedure and defer the insertion of the prosthesis until there is good healing of the incisions. This decision will depend on the tension of the closure and, to a major extent, on the innate conservatism of the surgeon. To date, we have not had to delay or stage the procedure, and have encountered neither flap slough nor extrusion of the implant through a broken-down incision. Figure 6-6A and B shows the preoperative status and postoperative result of the foregoing procedure. Figure 6-7A and B shows a similar result in a bilateral case.

After reconstruction has been completed and the operative site allowed to settle down, two further options need to be considered by the patient and her surgeon. The breasts will in all probability be somewhat asymmetric, raising the question of an equalizing procedure on the contralateral breast (usually a ptosis correction or reduction mammaplasty) (Fig. 6-8). This should also be discussed with the referring general surgeon, who, in situations where contralateral disease is statisti-

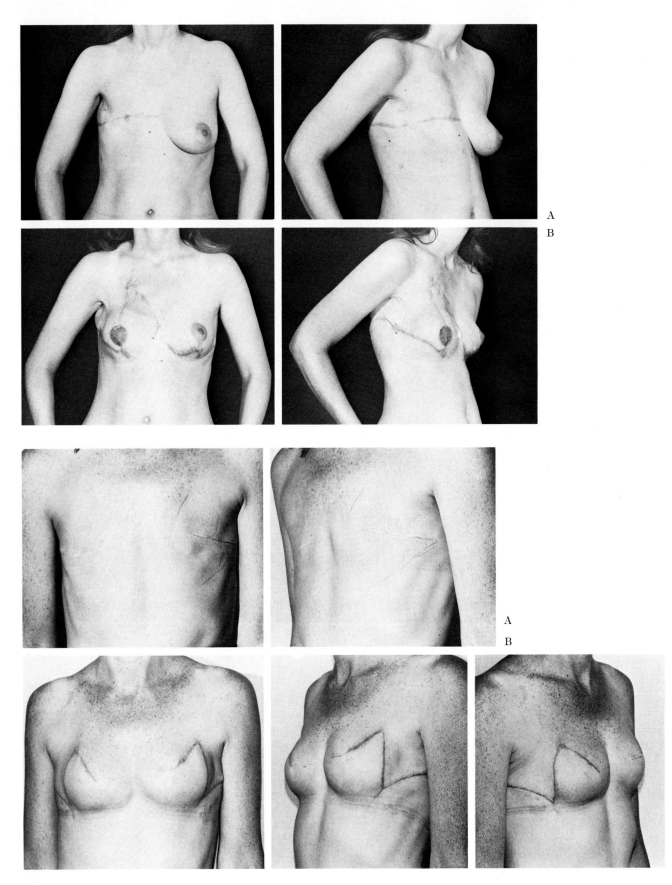

A

B

A

B

◄ FIG. 6-6.

A. A well-healed horizontal scar from a modified radical mastectomy performed two years previously. B. Following reconstruction with transposition flap and simultaneous augmentation. Elevation of the slightly ptotic opposite side and labial graft to the nipple have also been accomplished.

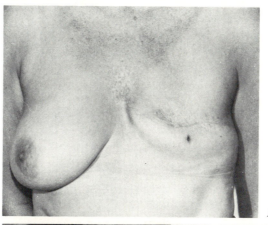

A

◄ FIG. 6-7.

A. A case of bilateral modified radical mastectomy with horizontal incision. B. Reconstructed with transposition flaps and implants. Nipple reconstruction was not requested.

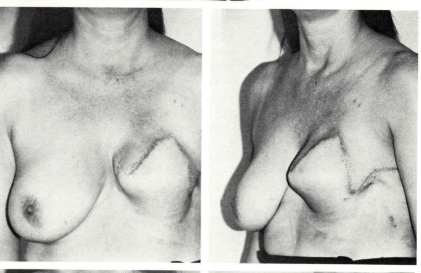

B
C

FIG. 6-8.

A. Healed modified radical mastectomy. B. Reconstruction with a transposition flap and implant. Marked asymmetry. C. Reasonable symmetry is accomplished by reducing the hypertrophic and ptotic opposite breast.

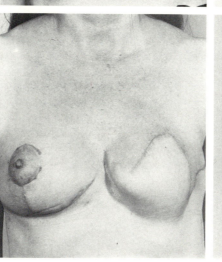
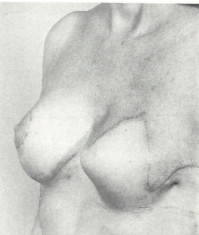

cally likely, may request a prophylactic subcutaneous mastectomy.

Construction of a nipple may be important to some patients, although the majority are happy with a satisfactorily restored breast contour as described. If requested this may be accomplished by Millard's split-thickness graft from the opposite nipple,[14] Cronin's nipple-sharing procedure,[5] or, as we prefer, a free composite graft from the labium minor.

Vertical Scar

A vertical scar is generally employed in the standard radical mastectomy, which operation presents a far more difficult problem of reconstruction for three reasons (Fig. 6-9).

1. With sacrifice of the pectoral musculature, there is a marked contour deficiency below the clavicle—an area frequently exposed by most modes of dress.
2. The skin flaps are both thinner and generally closed under greater tension than with the modified radical mastectomy. Thus, the closure over a prosthesis is less secure and requires, almost without exception, the addition of more tissue to the anterior thorax.
3. There is no delay phenomenon as produced by the horizontal incision, and the blood supply to the medially based (and therefore retrograde) flap will depend entirely on the inferior epigas-

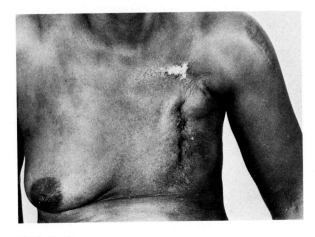

FIG. 6-9.
A typical healed radical mastectomy. Note tight skin cover and depigmentation following irradiation.

tric and external iliac vessels together with the thoraco-epigastric anastomosis.

However, a medially based interpolation flap may be employed to provide the tissue necessary for secure coverage of any implant. Even greater care must be taken in the design and transfer of the flap than described in the previous section, because the flap will need to be larger (to replace a much greater tissue deficit) and is inherently less viable from a vascular standpoint.

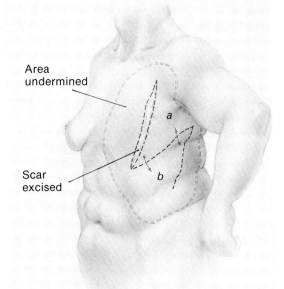

Area undermined

Scar excised

a

b

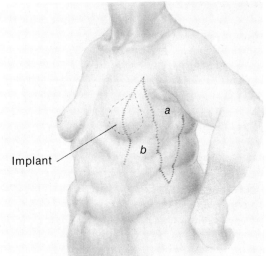

Implant

a

b

II-1

II-2

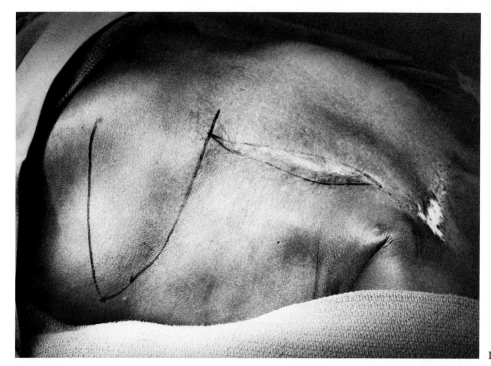

II-3

II-4

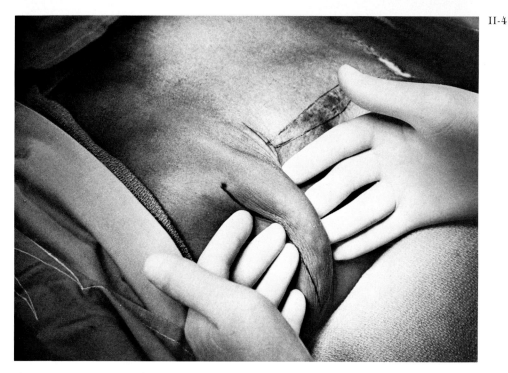

Again, an asymmetric Z-plasty is planned (II-1, II-2). The vertical scar is excised (II-3), and, with medial and lateral undermining, the adjacent tissue is allowed to spring apart. This now represents the upper limb of the Z. A large medially based flap is planned (II-4) with a horizontal upper edge, and a lower edge is cut obliquely from the tip of the flap to the umbilicus (II-5).

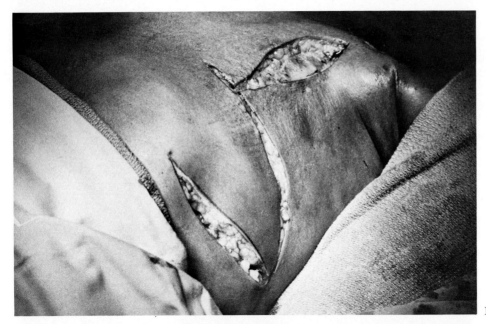

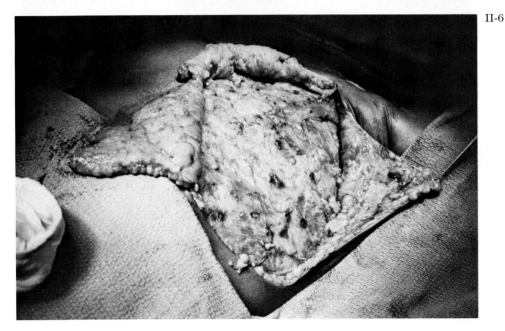

The length of the flap is predetermined by how far it needs to reach the axilla or clavicle; the width will depend on the skin deficit to be closed loosely enough to provide room for a suitable implant. This flap should rarely, if ever, be cut according to eye judgment; preplanning with a template in the dimensions of the tissue deficit and rotated to the proposed flap site is virtually mandatory.

The flap, due to its location and dimensions, will frequently require a delay. This should be explained to the patient prior to the procedure. In addition, the undermining required to mobilize the flap and achieve closure of the secondary defect is quite extensive—to the posterior axillary line laterally, to the iliac crest and inguinal ligament inferiorly, and across the midline medially. Failure to undermine widely will lead to closure under too much tension.

170

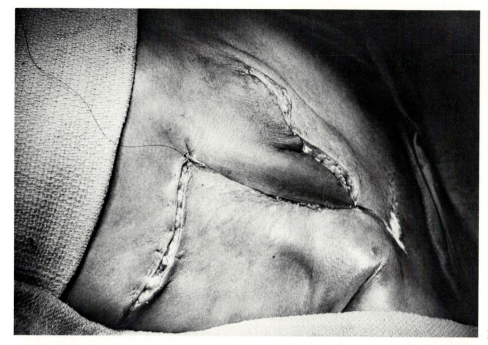

II-7

II-8

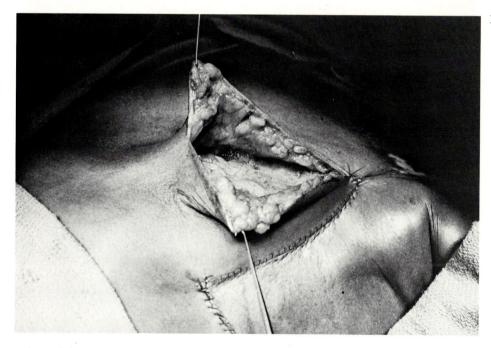

A useful maneuver at the time of flap transfer is to de-epithelialize the tip of the flap for a variable distance and bury it beneath the infraclavicular skin. This will serve not only to reinforce the closure but also to fill in the hollow referred to previously.

Once the flap transfer has been completed satisfactorily (II-6, II-7) (either as a single procedure or staged), the question arises as to whether or not to proceed with simultaneous augmentation (II-8, II-9, II-10).

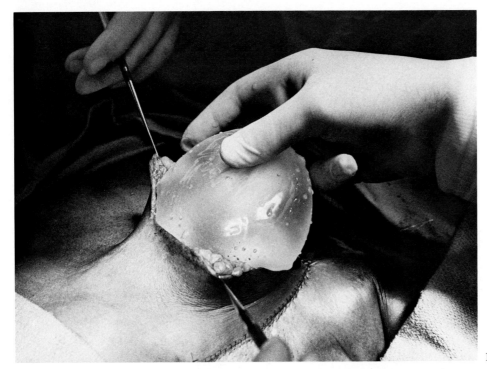

II-9

II-10

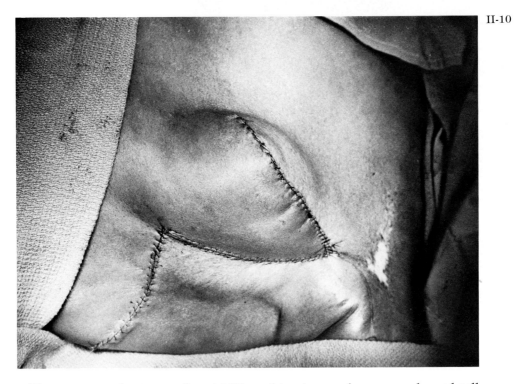

The same considerations—flap viability and tension on closure—apply, and call for a high degree of surgical judgment. Similarly, the later decisions dealing with contralateral breast reconstruction and creation of a nipple will be necessary.

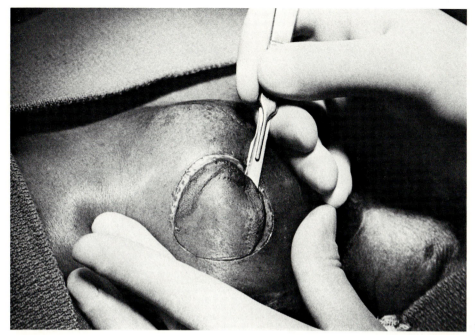

III-1

III-2

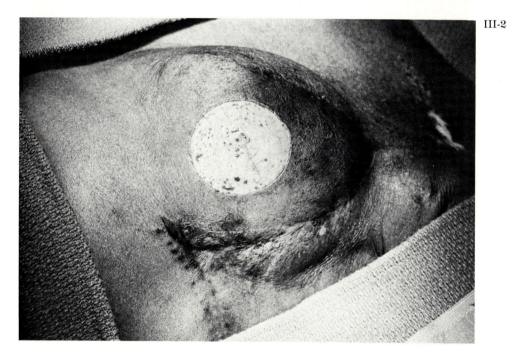

Reconstruction of the Nipple

As mentioned previously, our preferred method for reconstructing a nipple is by means of a labial full-thickness graft. Color and texture are a good match, and the donor site is hidden. A partial-thickness disk of skin, 5 cm. in diameter, is taken from the apex of the breast at a site matching the nipple on the opposite side (III-1), leaving dermis as a base for the labial graft (III-2).

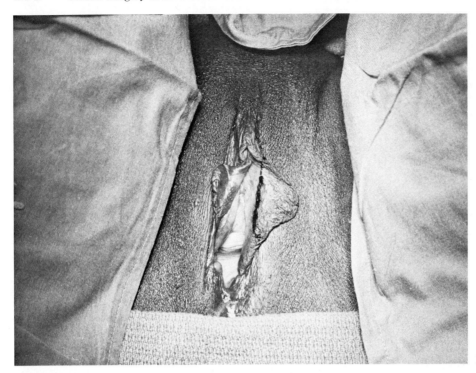

III-3

III-4

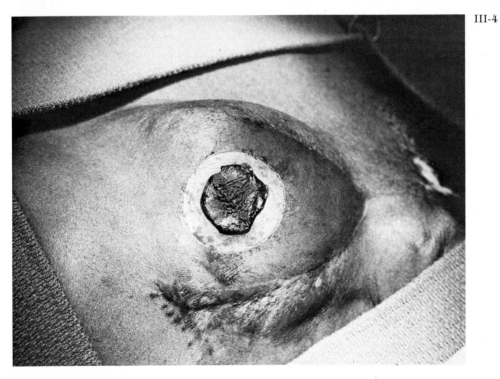

The graft is prepared by excising a circle of labium minor (III-3), minimally defatting and placing it on the prepared recipient site (III-4). It is then sutured in place with a conventional tie-over bolus dressing (III-5, III-6).

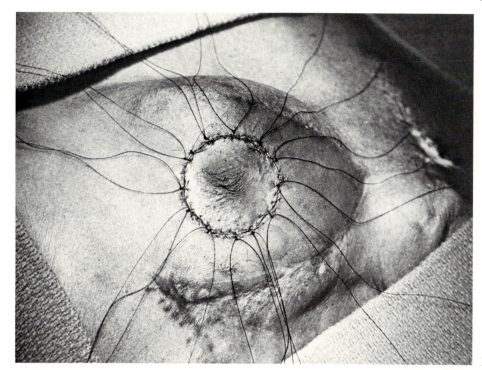

III-5

III-6

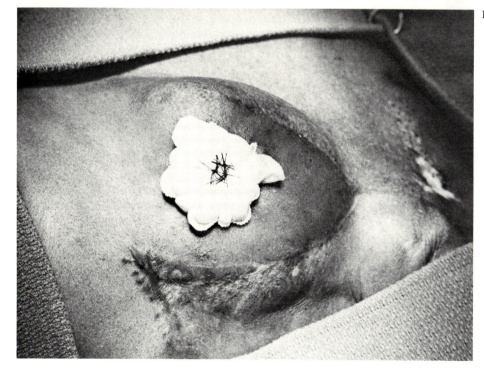

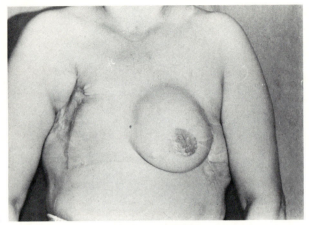

A

B

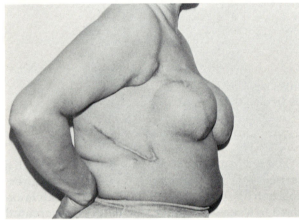

FIG. 6–13.
A. A difficult situation, involving bilateral radical mastectomies. Reconstruction on the left side had previously been attempted with indifferent results; the right side was left alone due to the tightness of the skin graft used for cover in the initial procedure. B. Following excision of the skin graft and interposition of a large enough flap to afford augmentation.

THE LATISSIMUS DORSI MYOCUTANEOUS FLAP

As mentioned earlier in this chapter, the latissimus dorsi muscle, frequently with its outerlying skin, can be used to reconstruct the breast and chest wall in those cases which demonstrate major skin and soft tissue deficit.

First described by D'Este in 1912,[6] this procedure was popularized by Olivari[17] and Muhlbauer,[16] and has been in widespread use in Europe for several years. More recently, McCraw,[13] Bostwick,[3] and Mathes and Nahai in an atlas of myocutaneous flaps[12] have described the procedure in all of its aspects in great detail.

ANATOMY

The latissimus dorsi muscle is a large triangular muscle with its base originating from the spinous processes of the seventh thoracic vertebra to the sacrum and posterior iliac crest. It picks up fleshy fibers originating from the lower three or four ribs and sometimes from the inferior angle of the scapula. The muscle inserts into the floor of the bicipital groove of the humerus and, near its insertion, helps to form the posterior axillary fold.

The arterial supply comes from the thoracodorsal artery, the termination of the subscapular artery. The thoracodorsal artery is accompanied by venae comitantes and the thoracodorsal nerve. The neurovascular bundle enters the deep surface of the muscle about 10 cm. from its insertion into the humerus.

Musculocutaneous perforators pierce the muscle to supply the overlying skin which can be fashioned into an island flap based transversely, obliquely, or longitudinally over the muscle. A secondary blood supply arises from the intercostal and lumbar arteries and enters the muscle near its vertebral origins.

The muscle is able to arc around its neurovascular pedicle in the posterior axillary fold and can reach defects in the lower lumbar, lateral chest, anterior chest, and upper arm regions.

INDICATIONS FOR THE USE OF A LATISSIMUS DORSI FLAP

The latissimus dorsi muscle simulates the pectoralis major muscle perfectly. It is therefore ideal for use in the reconstruction of the classical radical mastectomy defect. It provides well-padded coverage for an implant, and this cuts down on the high incidence of extrusion of the implant through the mastectomy scar or through the thin postmastectomy skin flaps.[13]

Reconstruction can safely be carried out in the postirradiated chest wall because the muscle brings with it its own adequate blood supply. It is therefore the method of choice in cases in which there is radionecrosis of the chest wall.

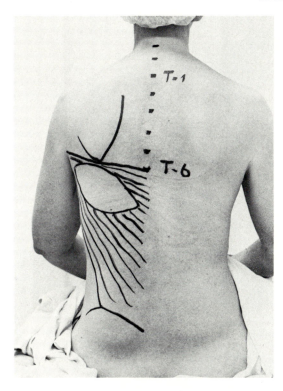

OPERATIVE TECHNIQUE

The landmarks of the latissimus dorsi muscle, the scapula, and the proposed size and situation of the skin island are accurately marked on the patient pre-operatively in the sitting position (IV-1). A cloth template should be cut with the proposed muscle and skin flap mapped out on it.

The posterior axillary fold is used as the rotation point. The template should rotate under the axilla and onto the front of the chest so as to allow the muscle to lie comfortably on the chest wall, substituting for the absent pectoralis major muscle. The skin island should then have the same size, shape, and orientation as the mastectomy scar and the defect created by releasing that scar. The donor wound can be closed primarily and will be hidden by the brassiere strap (IV-2).

The operation commences with the patient in the lateral position with the side to be reconstructed uppermost (IV-3).

IV-1

IV-2, IV-3

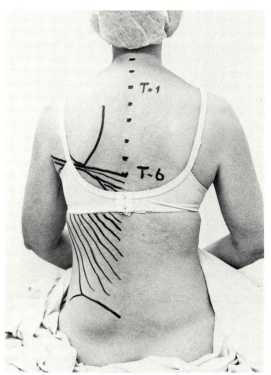

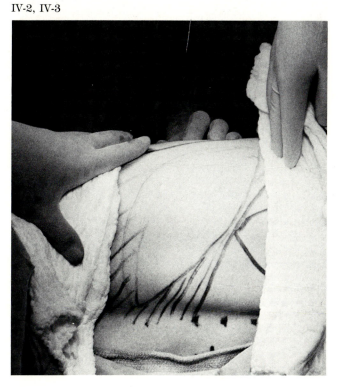

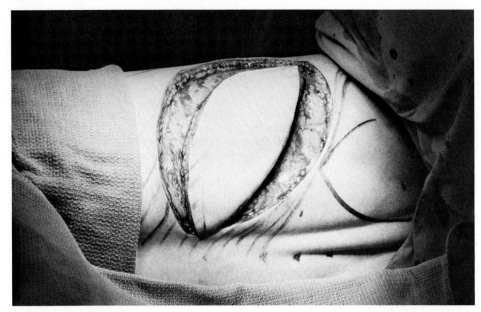

IV-4

IV-5

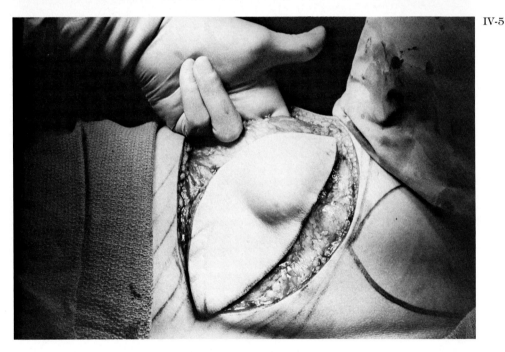

A two-team approach will save much time. The first team will raise the musculo-cutaneous flap while the second team prepares the anterior chest wall. The skin island is circumscribed with a scalpel down to the deep fascia covering the latissimus dorsi muscle (IV-4).

The anterolateral free border of the latissimus dorsi muscle is delineated and the deep aspect of the muscle is easily dissected free (IV-5). The superior free broder of the latissimus dorsi muscle is similarly dissected and detached from the inferior angle of the scapula. The muscle is then transected inferiorly (IV-6).

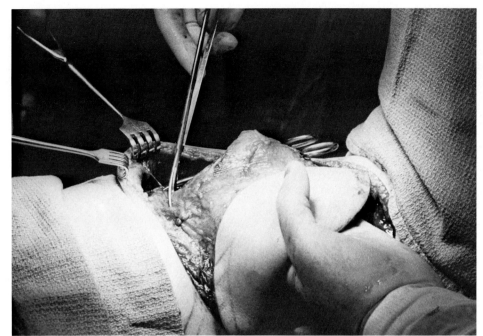

IV-6

IV-7

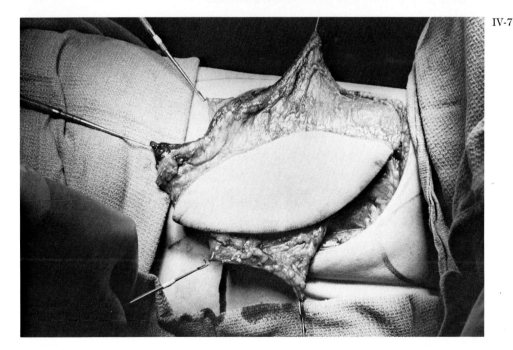

Mobilization of the muscle is completed by cutting its aponeurotic attachments medially as well as the deep fleshy fibers that originate from the lower three or four ribs. The medial perforating muscular vessels from the intercostal and lumbar vessels are ligated and divided.

The musculocutaneous flap is now free to rotate around the neurovascular hilum at the posterior axillary fold (IV-7). It is not necessary to visualize the neurovascular bundle which is situated on the deep surface of the muscle near its humeral insertion.

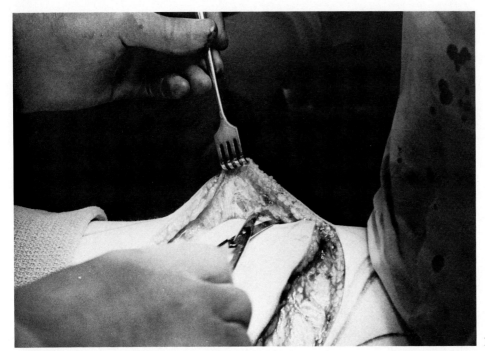

IV-8

IV-9

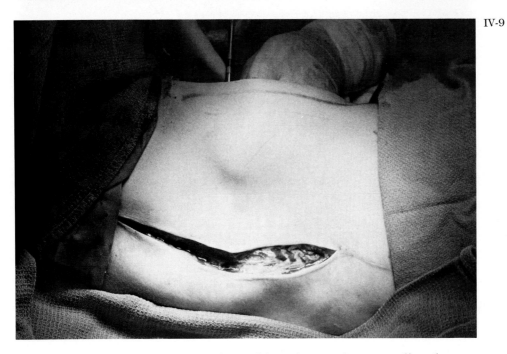

The skin over the lateral chest wall is widely undermined so as to allow the easy passage of the latissimus dorsi musculocutaneous flap onto the anterior aspect of the chest (IV-8). The undermining is directed forward toward the opened-up mastectomy scar (IV-9). The compound flap can now be delivered into the anterior chest wall defect (IV-10).

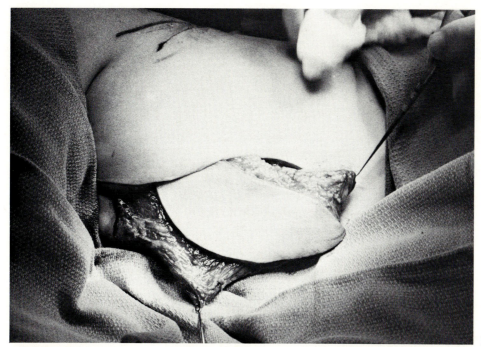

IV-10

IV-11

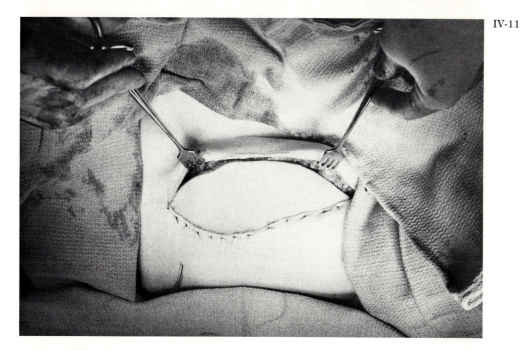

Meanwhile, the second team has been working simultaneously on the anterior aspect of the chest, opening up the mastectomy scar and undermining the skin widely, from the clavicle above to the ideal inframammary fold below, and from the sternum medially to meet the undermined lateral chest wall tunnel.

The lateral margin of the skin island is sutured to the lateral edge of the mastectomy wound and a drain is placed into the cavity (IV-11).

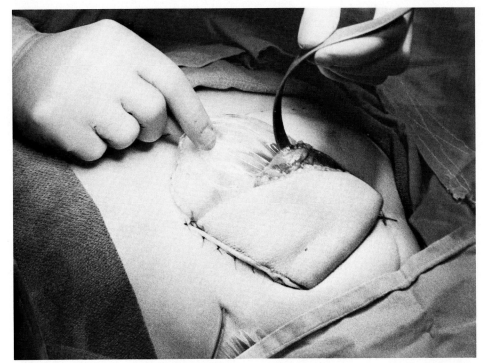

IV-12

IV-13

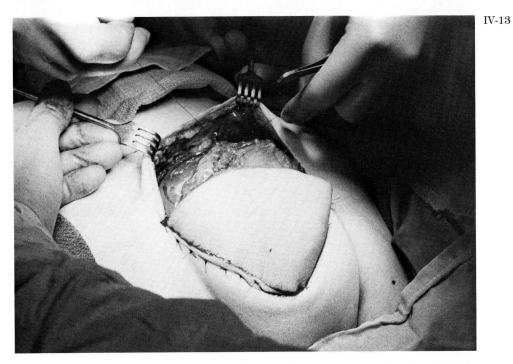

A suitably sized breast implant is placed behind the medial edge of the flap (IV-12). The medial edge of the latissimus dorsi muscle is sewn down to the sternal fascia (IV-13) and the pocket around the implant is carefully closed in order to keep the implant in its correct position (IV-14). If this is not done the implant may migrate into the axillary region.

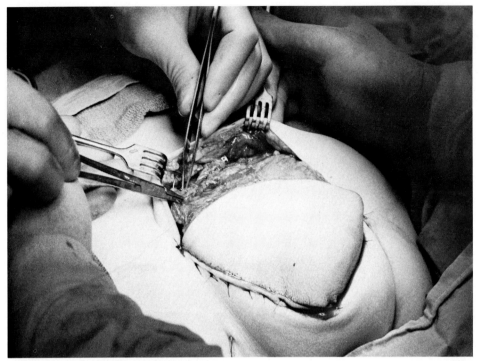

IV-14

IV-15

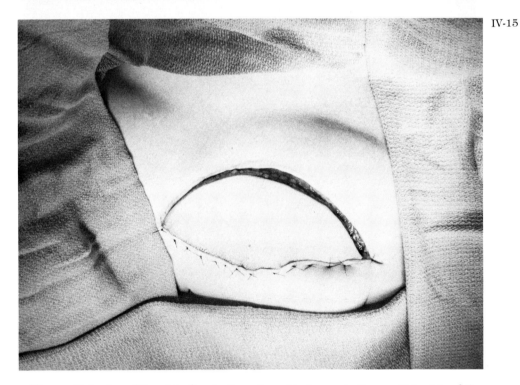

The medial edge of the skin flap is then closed in layers to the medial edge of the mastectomy scar (IV-15, IV-16), and the donor defect (IV-17) is closed in a linear fasion (IV-18).

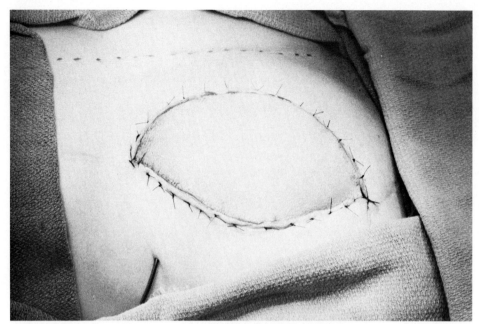

IV-16

IV-17

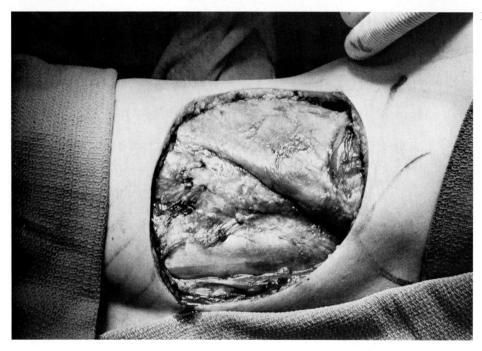

FIG. 6–14.
A. Preoperative views of the patient in the preceding se- ▶
quence, showing the tight scarring of the chest skin and
total absence of a breast mound. B. The reconstructed
breast, similar in bulk and contour to the contralateral
normal side, showing a well-healed and reasonably inconspicuous donor site scar.

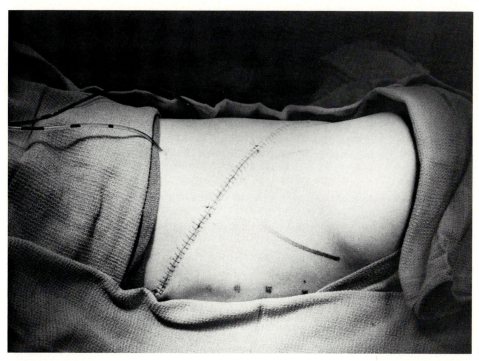

IV-18

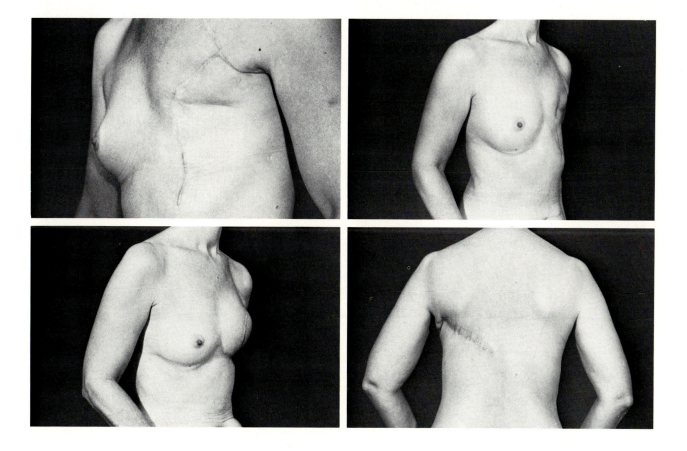

Pre- and postoperative views of the patient are shown in Figure 6-14A and B.

The last word has by no means been written on this dynamic topic. New and better reconstructive procedures are being devised just as greater understanding of cancer immunology is helping to tackle the heart of the problem. We hope that this chapter will be outdated by the time it is published but meanwhile feel happy to have been part of an effort which, we feel, is playing a distinct role in helping to alleviate the psychological devastation to all patients who sustain the loss of a breast.

REFERENCES

1. **Adams WM:** Free composite grafts of the nipples in mammaryplasty. South Surg J, 13:715, 1947

2. **Bohmert H:** Personal method for reconstruction of the female breast following radical mastectomy. Trans Int Congr Plast Surg, Paris, Masson, 1976

3. **Bostwick J, III, Nahai F, Wallace JF, Vasconez LO:** Sixty latissimus dorsi flaps. Plast Reconstr Surg 63:31, 1979

4. **Cocke W:** Breast Reconstruction Following Mastectomy for Carcinoma. Boston, Little, Brown, 1977

5. **Cronin TD, Upton J, McDonough JM:** Reconstruction of the breast after mastectomy. Plast Reconstr Surg 59:1, 1977

6. **D'Este S:** La technique de L'amputation de la mamelle pour carcinome mammaire. Rev Chir (Paris) 45:164, 1912

7. **Freeman BS:** Experiences in reconstruction of the breast after mastectomy. Clin Plast Surg 3:277, 1976

8. **Guthrie RH:** Breast reconstruction after radical mastectomy. Plast Reconstr Surg 57:14, 1976

9. **Hoehler H:** Reconstruction of the female breast after radical mastectomy. In Converse JM (ed): Reconstructive Plastic Surgery. Philadelphia, Saunders, 1977

10. **Hueston J, McKenzie G:** Breast reconstruction after radical mastectomy. Aust NZ Surg 9:161, 1976

11. **Hutchins EH:** A method for the prevention of elephantiasis. Surg Gynecol Obstet 69:795, 1939

12. **Mathes SJ, Nahai F:** In Clinical Atlas of Muscle and Musculocutaneous Flaps. St. Louis, CV Mosby, 1979, 363 pp.

13. **McCraw JB, Penix JO, Baker JW:** Repair of major defects of the chest wall and spine with latissimus dorsi myocutaneous flap. Plast Reconstr Surg 62:197, 1978

14. **Millard DR:** Breast reconstruction after radical mastectomy. Plast Reconstr Surg 58:283, 1976

15. **Mendelson BC, Masson JK:** Treatment of chronic radiation injury over the shoulder with a latissimus dorsi myocutaneous flap. Plast Reconstr Surg 60:681, 1977

16. **Muhlbauer W, Olbrisch R:** The latissimus dorsi myocutaneous flap for breast reconstruction. Chir Plastica 4:27, 1977

17. **Olivari N:** The latissimus flap. Br J Plast Surg 29:126, 1976

18. **Patey DH, Dyson WH:** The prognosis of carcinoma of the breast in relation to the type of operation performed. Br J Cancer 2:7, 1948

19. **Perras C:** The creation of a twin breast following radical mastectomy. Clin Plast Surg 3:265, 1976

20. **Snyderman RK, Guthrie RH:** Reconstruction of the female breast following radical mastectomy. Plast Reconstr Surg 57:14, 1976

21. **Urban JA:** Bilateral breast cancer. In Breast Cancer, Early and Late. Chicago, Yearbook Medical, 1970

7

psychiatric and legal implications of breast surgery

PSYCHOSOCIAL ASPECTS OF AUGMENTATION MAMMAPLASTY AND OF MASTECTOMY

RICHARD L. VANDENBERGH

AUGMENTATION MAMMAPLASTY

Society tends to determine our standards of desirability, not only in behavior but also in physical appearance. While some physical standards such as hair length seem to vary from generation to generation, or even every few months according to fashion, other physical factors seem relatively constant. For instance, the desirability of a slim and youthful physical appearance for women in our Western culture has lasted now for several generations. After the days of the flapper in the 1920s, the desirability of large breasts has been consistent. Every pinup, every young woman used to sell a product on television or a billboard has this attribute prominently displayed.

In addition, since the self-esteem of many women is dependent upon an acceptable physical appearance in society, the size of their breasts assumes paramount importance. In fact, many physically normal women develop an almost paralyzing self-consciousness focused on the feeling that they do not have the correct size bosom.

As if the above societal factors in and of themselves were not enough, it must also be remembered that the breast has been the symbol of femininity, motherhood, and feminine sexuality almost since man's beginning. The sight of the female breast is a stronger sexual stimulant for many males than the sight of the female genitalia. Breasts are sexual both in reality and symbolically. The breasts' importance as a symbol of motherhood is dramatically exemplified by the frequency of depression that occurs in women who feel that they have failed in their attempts at breast-feeding.

Plastic surgeons must keep all these factors in mind in dealing with their patients. For while many surgeons have no hesitation doing such corrective surgery as improvement of burn scars, dermabrasion of acne or traumatic facial scars, or correction of prominent ears in a young boy, they often do not sympathize with the woman who wants an augmentation mammaplasty. They seem to be oblivious to the fact that for many contemporary Western women, their feelings of sexual attractiveness, femininity, even general adequacy, are closely linked to an acceptable breast size. It is as if they fail to recognize that what is not important in their own self-concept is nevertheless extremely significant to many women. As long as the surgeon is capable of performing safe, successful operations, he should feel no basic reluctance to operate on the woman with breast problems.

THE SURGEON'S DILEMMA

Nevertheless, there are some specific factors which should make the surgeon reluctant to perform surgery and still others which contraindicate surgery.

Previous reports clearly indicate that augmentation mammaplasty has met with both success and failure. It should be remembered by the cosmetic surgeon that the desired operative changes are designed to allow the patient to conform more closely to the aesthetic standards of her social group—that is, to merge with the crowd—but not to become some latter-day Venus or Marilyn Monroe.[8] The average profile of the woman seeking augmentation mammaplasty reveals a white, married housewife, of middle socioeconomic class, with one or more children, an age range of 22 to 42 (with a mean of 30 to 31), no particular religious affiliation, and a chronically low self-esteem in regard to her breasts and general body image.[2] Studies of the patients' personalities have indicated that, while they are all different kinds of people, there are also discernible factors that they have in common. Almost every patient has experienced serious difficulties in her mother-daughter relationship.[4] They demonstrate a chronic low self-esteem, often dating back to puberty, which even when previously worked through psychiatrically is frequently rekindled postpartum. Hysterical characteristics and a higher than usual concern for their appearance are not uncommon, and some see their small breasts as punishment for having sexual feelings directed toward their fathers. Often underlying the chronic low self-esteem is an equally chronic depression.

In many of these cases, the patient's husband has been informed, and he usually does not feel the operation is necessary. The husband in most cases reassures the patient that he already considers the patient's breasts adequate and attractive. The patient, however, frequently either does not believe her husband, or does not care particularly if her husband is against the operation. Most patients are determined to have the operation in the face of any obstacles, and the surgeon will frequently note a sense of urgency in their demands.

Previous studies with patient samples similar to the above have revealed both predictable and less predictable results. Predictably, those patients who postoperatively experience severe hardening, chronic infections, problems with drainage, or other surgical complications are universally disappointed. They say such things as "I should never have been so stupid," or "I should have known this would happen to me." Such self-depreciatory remarks fit with the patient's already-existing low self-esteem. Frequently these patients will regress and withdraw as a result of this real disfigurement.

Equally predictable is the fact that those patients who have undergone surgically successful operations experience such positive results as an improved self-image, increased social ease, decreased self-consciousness, improved sexual relations and enjoyment, and a decreased fixation on their breasts. Furthermore, their breast fixation has not been followed by a transfer fixation onto any other replacement object. Many women experience and describe even more widespread positive psychiatric and social results. They report that, along with their improved self-esteem, they are truly happy for the first time in their lives. Motherhood becomes far more enjoyable and their children no longer seem an imposition on their lives. In these successful surgical cases, negative psychiatric sequelae have been far less common than originally feared. Follow-up studies of 4, 10, and 12 years show that the vast majority of patients are happy with their results.[3]

The surgeon's dilemma appears in those cases which demonstrate unpredictable results. Some patients will express delight and satisfaction over results considered mediocre by the surgeon. But of much more concern are those patients without any disfigurement who complain bitterly following anatomically near-perfect reconstruction. While the other chapters of this book describe primarily how technically to achieve surgical success, this chapter will concentrate on how to reduce to a minimum the number of those patients who, after physically successful results, nonetheless remain emotionally bitter, disappointed, and depressed.

This is truly the cosmetic surgeon's dilemma. The surgeon must learn how to exclude in advance those patients who will derive no benefit from successful surgery, who will remain chronically dissatisfied and therefore will badger for further corrections, who will suffer major psychiatric breakdowns, or who will even take the surgeon to court over the positive results of the surgery. At the same time, in attempting to avoid this dilemma, the surgeon must not become overly cautious and thereby exclude partially neurotic and depressed individuals who would greatly benefit in many aspects of their lives from successful surgery.

CRITERIA FOR SELECTION
Positive Indications

All women requesting augmentation mammaplasty present themselves with physical, emotional, and social complaints. The surgeon's task is to separate the "legitimate complaints," those based largely on reality and therefore likely to be helped by successful surgery, from those based on delusion and unrealistic expectations. There are common categories which can be used to classify those women presenting with "legitimate" complaints.

The first category consists of small-breasted or flat-chested women. These are often housewives with several children who have been self-conscious about their breast size for years and who postpartum have lost much of the little breast development they previously possessed. Often a degree of ptosis is associated with the hypoplasia. Although their husbands may deny any conscious unhappiness, they nonetheless simultaneously make unfavorable comments, overtly or by implication, comparing the patient's breast size to those of other women among their friends, acquaintances, or women on the television or movie screen. The realistic smallness of these women's breasts is repugnant to them and, even if their husbands are genuinely content, the women themselves feel unattractive and consequently disinclined toward sex in general and sex play with their breasts in particular. Some women in this category have jobs which expose them to frequent teasing from men. Restaurant and cocktail waitresses are common examples; others are divorced or separated women who feel that an augmentation mammaplasty will increase their chances of attracting a new potential partner. One of the most important clues to a positive prognosis for women in this category is their primary desire to gratify their own egos and improve their own self-images. They are far less concerned about how the augmentation will affect others, including their husbands. These women often state that they feel "empty inside," "inadequate," "hollow," "unacceptable to themselves," and that it is an internal, not an external, problem. The use of any external devices such as padded bras or falsies is unacceptable. They wish the artificial device to be implanted underneath the skin, for only then can it become incorporated as part of their body image. Comparatively, the external devices are considered "phony" and "cheating." It must be stressed that the motivation for many of the women in this group is life-long intrapsychic doubts about their own femininity. It is their private and not their public image that counts. Most, if asked, will admit that they want the surgery even if they are to live alone on a desert island for the rest of their lives.

A second category of women seeking augmentation, and who have a good prognosis, consists of professional women such as entertainers and exotic dancers. These are women who have small breasts in comparison to their competition and they are realistically motivated by the demands and expectations of their profession.

A third, but small, group of women who seek augmentation consists of those with asymmetry in such forms as hypoplasia or aplasia of one breast. This group of patients has uniformly been among the most grateful and happy with the results of achieving breast symmetry.

Contraindications

The busy cosmetic surgeon does not have time to do a complete psychiatric history, but the use of a brief screening interview which touches on the following points will help to distinguish those patients who need more in-depth questioning. The following factors are indicators of poor emotional and social prognosis following augmentation mammaplasty.

1. The patient's motivation for the surgery appears to come largely externally from others important in her life. In addition, she expects the surgery to produce immediate and miraculous positive changes in the attitudes of these others toward her.

2. The patient is vague when trying to describe the exact reconstruction that she is seeking. At the same time, the size, shape, and symmetry of her breasts appear within normal limits. The surgeon should be cautioned here, however, not to use too rigid or absolute or so-called scientific measurements such as the patient's height, weight, and bone structure to determine what is normal breast size, for it is the patient's internal concept of breast inadequacy that she is striving to correct.[1]

3. The patient has derived and enjoyed a large amount of secondary gain from her small breasts. For example, she has used them as excuses in such varied areas as social, interpersonal, and career failures, and sexual avoidance or inactivity.

4. If the timing of the surgical request is tied into some major life crisis to which augmentation mammaplasty would appear to have no logical connection (e.g., the death of a child), then delay of the surgery until some time after the crisis is over would be advisable.

5. A history of previous satisfactory operations for augmentation or other cosmetic surgery should always alert the surgeon to the possibility that the patient is what has previously been called an "insatiable" cosmetic surgery patient.[6]

6. The patient who demonstrates such a strong sense of urgency that she tries to tempt the surgeon into bypassing the usual and proper preoperative screening techniques should instead alert the surgeon into making a more in-depth evaluation before agreeing to surgery.

7. The history or presence of severe mental illness should be an extremely strong factor in considering surgery to be contraindicated. This would include such things as severe cancerphobia in a patient; a major depression; schizo-

phrenia; and the symptom of mental illness frequently seen in these patients—somatic delusions.[5]

The patients with somatic delusions deserve further discussion because they are frequently the ones who postoperatively, in spite of perfect surgical results, are dissatisfied. The dissatisfaction with the result becomes coupled with their general life-long dissatisfaction with their appearance and then gets displaced onto the surgeon, who subsequently may find himself with an unwarranted lawsuit on his hands.

Recognition of these patients, as with the insatiable cosmetic surgery patient, becomes all important because psychiatric treatment in these cases can be helpful whereas surgical intervention tends only to reinforce and crystallize the somatic delusion of physical deformity or inadequacy.

These patients are unfortunately not always easily recognizable, because often their delusion may be an encapsulated area of mental illness in an otherwise normal-appearing person. They may have an insignificant deformity which to them appears conspicuous or even normal-sized attractive breasts which to them appear ugly.

The following case history is an example:

C.F. was a 33-year-old unhappily married woman with one child, who sought revision of a previous augmentation mammaplasty after having had two previous operations, neither of which she felt left her satisfactorily large enough. The surgeon, however, felt that her breasts were significantly larger than average, symmetrical, soft, and that she had obtained an excellent surgical result.

In spite of this, the patient stated that her "small" breasts inhibited her from wearing many kinds of "sexy" clothes and bathing suits, and inhibited her from going to social events where she felt people always laughed at her flat-chestedness. She was also afraid to undress in front of her husband or have sex with him because she felt he found her unattractive.

Her history revealed that she had had a strong dominant mother with whom she had fought frequently and with whom she had made a poor feminine identification. Her father was both ineffectual and passive and occasionally subtley seductive toward her. She was a tomboy until later than most girls (16) and was athletic and comparatively muscular; she had had three minor homosexual experiences during her adolescence. The patient was extremely insecure about her femininity and ashamed and concerned about her latent homosexuality. Her breasts were, to her, the symbolic proof of her femininity, and it was as if she needed only to get them large enough

and they would then make up for her emotional insecurity and be an irrefutable denial of her homosexual tendencies.

In spite of the above, the patient appeared well-groomed, intelligent, and presented a logical and articulate argument as to why the third breast operation should be carried out. She also flattered the surgeon, telling him that she had heard he was the best plastic surgeon in the country and that she had total confidence in his ability to succeed where the others had failed.

As in this case, a somatic delusion is often designed unconsciously to fill an emotional need or an unrecognized gap in the patient's self-esteem. There are unrealistic, almost magical expectations, as with this patient who expected the surgery to remove her fears of homosexuality along with her inhibitions in sex with her husband. She was looking for an external cure for major internal conflicts.

The surgeon should also remember that somatic delusions are frequently associated with schizophrenia. Therefore, when the surgeon perceives a possible delusion, reinforcing evidence in the patient's history suggestive of a lonely, isolated life style should be looked for. Again, it must be emphasized that the somatic delusion may be present in an otherwise normal-appearing patient.

HOW, WHEN, AND IF TO USE A PSYCHIATRIST

How, when, and if to use a psychiatrist depends to a large extend upon the individual personality and practice of the cosmetic surgeon. If the surgeon has the time to do in-depth interviewing with those of his patients who need it, if he feels comfortable listening to and dealing with these patients' emotions, and, finally, if he feels he has sufficient skill and knowledge in this area, the use of a psychiatrist becomes restricted to the rare case.

There seems little question that the rapport between the surgeon and the patient is of paramount importance. If the surgeon has the time, capabilities, and interest, then this represents the best possible solution. Unfortunately, a thorough understanding of a patient's motivation for surgery requires a truly time-consuming interview, including such factors as the patient's past mental history, the nature of her family and peer relationships, her psychosexual development, the patient's methods and abilities for coping with stress, the patient's personal attributes, the reasons behind the timing of the request for surgery, the implications of the surgery for the patient, plus any other avenues of inquiry which might be indicated during the course of the interview (e.g., current life crises).

There are many surgeons who are reluctant to be cast into what they consider to be the role of a psychiatrist with a knife. In such cases, it is frequently useful for the surgeon to have a regular working arrangement with a local psychiatrist who will be available for all his psychiatric referrals. This enables the psychiatrist to gain experience and expertise in this specialized area, and yields more accurate, consistent assessments and allows follow-up studies to refine decision-making and possibly to design further research studies.

The timing and method in which the referral is made are also of prime importance. The surgeon must not be ambivalent about the use of a psychiatrist and therefore about referrals. Ambivalence on the part of the surgeon is quickly picked up by the patient, and since many of these patients much prefer to see themselves as having physical deformities or inadequacies, the chances of them ever showing up for their appointment with the psychiatrist are not good. The surgeon must be firmly positive as well as tactful in the manner in which the psychiatric evaluation is suggested.

For instance, the patient who is told "Perhaps you should see a psychiatrist before we proceed any further. That might make you a little more confident about what you're doing. I can't promise it will help, but it certainly can't do you any harm, so I think you should give it a try" will never keep the first appointment. Rather, the surgeon should stress that psychiatric evaluation will benefit the patient, that it is extremely important for a positive outcome, and that it is not being done because the patient is "mentally ill" but for general help in adjusting to what will be an important change in her physical appearance and body image.

Sometimes the patient is afraid that if she does not impress the psychiatrist positively she will be refused the operation. She may then attempt to put on a facade for the psychiatrist by trying to second guess what he wishes to hear. The patient should be reassured that the psychiatric interview is not a test that one can pass or flunk.

In fact, the surgeon and psychiatrist team has several options to offer the patient. First, a psychiatric referral is more likely to be successful pre-operatively rather then postoperatively. Surgery can be withheld temporarily while psychiatric evaluation is carried out, and can be held out as the real but future carrot to help motivate the patient until the completion of her psychotherapy. Similarly, the patient in the middle of a life crisis (e.g., divorce) can be told that surgery should be delayed and appropriate psychotherapy received until she has an opportunity to step back from the disturbing external environmental circumstances and gain some objectivity on her life.

Psychotherapy need not be restricted in timing. It can take place before surgery, in conjunction and simultaneously with surgery, postoperatively, or any combination of the above. The patient who is willing to begin indicated psychotherapy pre-operatively frequently demonstrates by this willingness alone that she has some insight and objectivity on the emotional aspects of her problem, that her delusions and bodily preoccupations (when present) are less likely to be totally fixed or unalterable, and that her prognosis is better.

Psychotherapy can offer support for the fragile patient when used in conjunction with the surgery. Similarly, it can facilitate postoperative improvement and decrease the likelihood of postoperative depression.

It should be remembered and emphasized here that these patients frequently use denial and repression before their surgery. Such denial of the risks and complications of surgery may be a major reason for many of the unfounded legal suits. For this reason alone, augmentation mammaplasty should never be presented to the patient in the initial interview as the "only desirable" solution to her problems, and the possible complications of surgery should, if anything, be overstressed. All patients should be told that all is not yet known concerning the long-range effects of implants and that further knowledge may lead to the recall and possible removal of the implants. It may be advisable not to operate on any patient unwilling to accept this possibility.

Finally, it should be mentioned that frequently these patients will simply not accept psychiatric referral no matter how positively and tactfully it is presented. Instead, a patient may shop from one surgeon to another until she finds that surgeon who will operate in spite of her emotional problems and who will end up with the brunt of the patient's psychosis or delusional system on his hands—in or out of court.

EMOTIONAL SEQUELAE OF AUGMENTATION MAMMAPLASTY

Frequently, there is a transient acute emotional disturbance seen in the immediate postoperative period. This may consist of a few minutes to several days of weepy outbursts, frequent sense of embarrassment, and frequent self-scrutiny and self-handling, all of which are the patient's attempts to integrate her new body image tactiley, visually, and emotionally. Understanding and some psychological reinforcement and praise are all that is needed for remission of these symptoms.

In attempting to assess postoperative results, it should always be kept in mind that the patient may be hesitant to express minor disappointments to the surgeon on whom she may still feel dependent and toward whom she may feel great gratitude. It must be remembered that the patient's communication with her doctor is often influenced by what she perceives or needs her relationship with him to be. In spite of this, it should be stressed that following technically successful surgery the patient's feelings were positive in the vast majority of cases. Patients' reports include a whole range of positive reactions. Many say that once they lose their breast-centered orientation and embarrassment they become more confident and comfortable in low-cut clothes and bathing suits. Whether their husbands express relative indifference or pleasure with their new breast size, the patients themselves express heightened sexual desire and desirability. Sexual intercourse itself is reported as being subjectively more satisfying, and several patients have stated that they have experienced orgasm for the first time in their lives. Those who admitted phobic anxiety or repugnancy about being touched on the breasts preoperatively reported the disappearance of this feeling postoperatively.

As indicated previously in this chapter, the postoperative personality changes extended into many areas of these patients' lives. They felt generally more confident, less peculiar, and as good as other women at last. They felt that any pathologic jealousy of other women was significantly reduced. Many turn to activities of a more extroverted nature. The ability to give to their children and to enjoy the demands of motherhood was increased.

Many husbands noted increased happiness in their wives and improved attitudes and moods.

Sometimes patients are tempted to misuse their new-found sense of freedom from sexual and other inhibitions, as well as their new sense of self-confidence and attractiveness, to become involved in what prove to be unfortunate relationships. Patients should, of course, be warned of this danger. However, the overriding impression of the psychosocial results of a successful augmentation mammaplasty can perhaps best be summed up by those women who say "I only wish I had had the operation years ago."

MASTECTOMY

In the introduction to augmentation mammaplasty, the importance of the breast to a woman was discussed in its many different aspects. However, when the surgery being considered is removal of the breast rather than correction of size or assymetry, several crucial additional factors must be considered. The overriding factor is the patient's need to deal not only with the loss of a breast but also the possible ensuing loss of life from cancer. Although the patient, particularly if the cancer has been detected and reported early, may be a long time away from dying, she may still see herself as having a fatal disease. All the emotions involved in truly confronting one's own mortality for the first time will then have been internally aroused.

Even if the patient can be convinced that she is not in imminent danger of losing her life, she must still face the acute loss of her breast, which (as we have discussed) is such an emotionally invested part of a woman's body and body image. Additionally, the appearance of the human body often plays a significant role in determining the individual's style for social and sexual interaction. Its continuity in time is closely bound up with a person's sense of a stable identity. A sudden change of appearance may disrupt this feeling of self-continuity and lead to feelings of panic, depersonalization, confusion, and depression.

The woman must also for the first time face all the emotional problems surrounding deformity. In the animal world a damaged or deformed member of a species is likely to be rejected or even overtly attacked by the rest. Unfortunately, human society has many parallels in the case of a disfigured person. Perhaps the most famous are Quasimodo in

Victor Hugo's **The Hunchback of Notre Dame** and Long John Silver in Robert Louis Stevenson's **Treasure Island**. But even the lesser-known villains of many movies are frequently distinguished by large scars disfiguring their faces or a deformed hand or missing finger. The postmastectomy woman must cope not only with her disfigurement but also with frequent reminders of its presence when she bathes, dresses, looks in the mirror, or makes love.

A final major distinction between an augmentation mammaplasty and a mastectomy is the latter's nonelective nature. As a result, the woman faced with a mastectomy often feels trapped and helpless. She may feel she is being punished for some real or imagined sin she may have at one time committed. Therefore, she often experiences a sense of guilt and subsequent depression. Or she may feel that she has always been a "good woman," and then asks "why me?" and feels a great sense of injustice and anger that is difficult to express or direct appropriately.

Additionally distressing are the reports in the literature and the numerous reports from patients themselves that the surgeon frequently has a tendency either to downplay the woman's feelings or to neglect or deny their importance. Such reactions are particularly puzzling in view of the fact that breast cancer is the commonest cancer in women, that numerous articles have been written on this subject, and that there are several self-help organizations started by the women themselves, thereby emphasizing their own recognition of need for emotional support and understanding.

THE SURGEON'S DILEMMA

Once again, as with augmentation mammaplasty, if the surgeon is as comfortable in dealing with the patient's emotions as he is in wielding his scalpel, he is the best possible person to do so. The patient almost always starts off with a positive transference toward her surgeon. She is forced to place her trust in him. She becomes by necessity first and by desire second to depend on him as her lifesaver. She sees him as capable of curing both her physical and emotional ills, and she transfers almost godlike powers onto him, which can be an extremely positive force in supporting the patient through all the stages of mastectomy.

Unfortunately, the surgeon is frequently ambivalent about this role, and with good reasons.[7] His caseload is often such that he does not have the time to spend on lengthy psychotherapeutic sessions pre- and postoperatively. Furthermore, many surgeons feel that if they become too immersed in the psychological as well as the surgical aspects of all their mastectomy patients, it might be at the cost of their own emotional stability. Finally, many surgeons feel that by probing too deeply they will open Pandora's box and not be equipped either with the time or knowledge to handle what emerges.

Nevertheless, the surgeon is always forced to play the role of the psychiatrist to some degree because the patients will either ask emotionally laden questions of him, or present themselves to him with spoken or unspoken demands for psychological support and understanding. For the surgeon who wishes only to deal with these questions and expectations there are guidelines which will be covered in the following sections.

PREOPERATIVE CONSIDERATIONS

The interval between the initial discovery of the lump and the results of the biopsy can be one of extreme anxiety and stress. The patient's fears and fantasies tend to run amok, frequently fed by myth and ignorance. The importance of this time period psychologically should not be underestimated. The surgeon who does not feel he can become more than peripherally involved in the psychological aspects should begin at this point to muster other sources of emotional support for the patient.

First, he should acknowledge to the patient his awareness that this can be a frightening and stressful occurrence in her life and, therefore, suggest to her that while he realizes that she is not "mentally ill," many women find it beneficial to receive emotional support from a psychiatrist during this period. Perhaps one of the major indicators of the high degree of stress engendered in a woman by the discovery of a breast lump is the finding by one group of researchers that 10 per cent of women waited three months between the time of the discovery and reporting it to a physician.[10]

The areas that a psychiatrist (or the surgeon if he so chooses) should cover in preoperative interviews with the patient include providing information to the patient about the various steps she will have to undergo. Once the need for a mastectomy is definite, the patient should be reassured that crying spells or some kind of mourning should not only be expected but are natural and healthy. The timing of the operation should be carefully explained to eliminate any chance of misconception. For instance, the uninformed patient who has to wait a few days for her operation may incorrectly conclude either that there is no hurry because it is already too late and the cancer has spread or that there is no hurry because her type of cancer is less serious. In fact, as much information about the procedure and postoperative procedures as possible should be explained to the patient. The physician must walk the difficult line between, on the one hand, not presenting the patient with so much information that an unnecessarily pessimistic prognosis is painted and, on the other hand, not giving false assurances where no definite future can be guaranteed. To guard against such mishaps in communication, the surgeon should always attempt to discuss with everyone involved in the patient's treatment (the nurse, the intern, the resident, etc.) exactly what she has been, is, and will be told. Inconsistent communication from different members of the treatment team is a major source of stress for the patient. Similarly, experience has shown that lying to the patient leads in the long run to anger, suspicion, and then distrust of the truth when it is finally told. A relatively small percentage of patients fail to adjust reasonably well to the truth after the initial period of upset and shock. In cases in which the husband has been told the truth while the patient has not, the latter ends up distrusting both husband and surgeon. The surgeon should be wary of the husband (or any other relative) who wants to establish a secret collusion with him.

Another area to be discussed in the preoperative interview with the patient should be what she will tell the significant people in her life about her situation.

After the patient has been appropriately informed, she should be given ample opportunity to ask questions so that any unforeseen fears or misconceptions can also be rapidly dispelled. Many physicians would like to find some definitive successful method for approaching these patients' psychological problems and then consistently use that method. Consequently, in practice many physicians are inflexible where a varied approach depending on the specific and changing needs of the individual patient is called for.

In addition to the psychiatrist, the surgeon can frequently turn to the husband to provide further emotional support for the patient. The husband will be most useful when he feels that his views have been considered important and of value to the surgeon from the time of the tumor's discovery throughout the postoperative period.

Female nurses can also play a key role in providing emotional support since frequently women feel freer in discussing some crucial problem areas with members of their own sex. The ideal situation exists when a female psychiatric liaison nurse is available who can follow the patient from the preoperative clinic through the rehabilitation period.

POSTOPERATIVE CONSIDERATIONS

This discussion will not consider the physical rehabilitation of the postmastectomy patient beyond saying that where the surgeon during postoperative visits asks his patient how she is doing she will often answer "fine," assuming that he is inquiring solely about her physical progress. The surgeon should avoid such a general question or not be lulled by such an answer into assuming that the total rehabilitation of his patient is progressing well. This discussion will concentrate instead on the cosmetic and emotional rehabilitation of the patient.

Aesthetic rehabilitation is an area in which the need for an individualized approach to each patient is most apparent. While information concerning breast reconstruction given immediately postoperatively or even preoperatively will be psychologically encouraging to some patients, it will be received by others as an indication of insensitivity and coldness on the part of the surgeon. To the patient who is still mourning the loss of her breast, still trying to reintegrate her self-image to the point of seeing herself as worthy once again of love and the rewards of life, and still adjusting to the fear of the possible recurrence of the cancer, talk of nipple grafting and breast reconstruction will be premature and poorly received. The surgeon must attempt to time his suggestions for aesthetic rehabilitation according to the individual patient's stage of emotional rehabilitation. If properly timed, a discussion on breast reconstruction can have dramatic positive effects on the patient's psyche.

The emotional rehabilitation of the patient involves several crucial areas. The immediate post-operative hospitalization period provides an excellent opportunity for the surgeon to talk naturally with the patient, her husband, and other important family members. This period can be used for primary prevention and secondary intervention. Various procedures can be discussed with the patient during this period, such as chemotherapy and radiotherapy. Again, as with the preoperative patient, the well-informed patient will handle (for instance) radiotherapy with far less stress than the ignorant patient who is prone to frightening fantasies and the half truths from the rumor mills.

Another important facet of rehabilitation that can be started during this period is the patient's acceptance of her disfigurement and scar. Since many patients postoperatively see their bodies as being disfigured and themselves as being "freaks" or "repugnant," and respond to this by refusing to look at their scar or allowing their husbands to see it for as long as possible, they should be helped and strongly encouraged while still in the hospital to look at, touch, and feel the area until it becomes less and less "strange" or "shocking." The husband should be similarly encouraged,[11] for although there is, of course, wide variation, some men do react to the first sight of the scar with shock and repugnance—a reaction that they can invariably overcome with time and familiarity.

The acceptance of the scar and the woman's new body shape by both herself and her husband is essential for their successful postoperative sexual relations. Even in the cases in which the husband finds the lack of one breast in no way repugnant and has no difficulty with his wife's scar, unless the woman finds herself sexually attractive her sexual drive and ability for sexual pleasure will diminish severely or disappear. Her ability to overcome her self-repugnance will be helped by positive sexual reactions and expressions of continued love, attraction, and a sense of romance on the part of her husband. He must be warned to avoid teasing or unsympathetic or insensitive criticism. He must be encouraged to reassure her while firmly refusing to allow her to avoid looking at her scar and sometimes insisting on sex even in the face of her unwillingness. But of equal if not greater importance will be the patient's ability to adjust emotionally to whatever symbolic loss of sexuality or femininity she herself attaches to the loss of her breast.

It should also be noted that some men, while not in any way repulsed by their wife's mastectomy, are nevertheless at a loss as to how to deal with it. Their confusion may be expressed by withdrawing from the situation, which in turn may be misinterpreted by the wife as sexual or other rejection.

Crucial to the woman's emotional rehabilitation is her ability to deal with the fact that the loss of a breast is a major psychological loss, and every major psychological loss that is dealt with emotionally in a healthy manner involves a period of bereavement or mourning. Mourning includes an initial shock or numbness, followed by a depressed affect and many of the symptoms and signs of depression, such as crying, social withdrawal, and difficulties with eating and sleeping. Mixed in with the depressed affect may be bitterness, resentment, and seemingly endless questioning protestations. Anger is also frequently seen, and may be directed at the staff, who in turn may take it personally out of ignorance. It is most important that the patient be encouraged to express her feelings concerning her loss. If instead the staff tries to "jolly" the patient along, her feelings will be suppressed and may come back to haunt her at a future date when she least needs it. It is for this precise reason that it is so important to inquire from the patient about any recent or remote past losses she has suffered and to garner whether those losses were adequately mourned. If such is not the case, the suppressed affect of the past losses will be added to the present loss of the breast and the patient's mourning will become a full-blown neurotic depression.

Neurotic depressions, including suicidal ideation, are frequently seen in postmastectomy patients in any case,[12] because these patients are already, by dint of their carcinoma, facing a potential second loss—the possible imminent loss of life. The fear of recurrence of their cancer (if not dealt with adequately) is constant. They are overly concerned with the possibility that some cancerous cells have been "left behind." They are supersensitive to every physical complaint and consequently are more prone to demonstrate "invalid" or repressed behavior.

Where there is a strong family history of breast cancer, the surgeon will frequently recommend to the woman that she soon undergo a further loss—the removal of her other breast. Many patients will unrealistically and dangerously refuse this second operation, but this is less likely to occur if they have been permitted and encouraged to mourn their first loss.

For those patients who do develop a neurotic depression, psychiatric care is definitely indicated.

Although some criticism has been voiced[9] regarding the use of personnel from such organizations as Reach to Recovery, it has been the author's experience that frequently these volunteers are most helpful, and when they are not, the patient will simply send them away. Similarly, the use of Prosthesis Clinics appears to be helpful for many patients.

A final area of importance is the education of the nurses on the surgical ward concerning the emotional needs and stresses of these patients. The uninformed nurse is more prone to be inappropriate in her approach and timing. The unwarned nurse is less likely to be aware that the patient with breast cancer forces her consciously or unconsciously to confront her own fears of breast cancer, mastectomy, and death. Such a confrontation may result in the nurse feeling unconsciously threatened by the patient and acting out this threat with unwitting hostility.

REFERENCES

1. **Edgerton MT, Mayer E, Jacobsen WE:** Augmentation mammoplasty. Psychiatric implications II. Further surgical and psychiatric implications. Plast Reconstr Surg 27:279, 1961

2. **Edgerton MT, McClary AR:** Augmentation mammoplasty. Plast Reconstr Surg 21:279, 1958

3. Cosmetic surgery of the breast (Roundtable discussion). Medical Aspects of Human Sexuality 6:4, 1970

4. **Druss RG:** Changes in body image following augmentation breast surgery. Int J Psychoanal Psychother 2:248, 1973

5. **Druss RG, Symonds FC, Crikelair GF:** The problem of somatic delusions in patients seeking cosmetic surgery. Plast Reconstr Surg 48:246, 1971

6. **Knorr NJ, Edgerton MT, Hooper JE:** The "insatiable" cosmetic surgery patient. Plast Reconstr Surg 40:285, 1967

7. **Asken MJ:** Psychoemotional aspects of mastectomy. Am J Psychiatry 132:56, 1975

8. **Olley PC:** Psychiatric aspects of cosmetic surgery. In Howells JG (ed): Modern Perspectives in the Psychiatric Aspects of Surgery. pp. 491–514. New York, Brunner-Mazel 1976

9. **McGuire P:** The psychological and social sequelae of mastectomy. In Howells JG (ed): Modern Perspectives in the Psychiatric Aspects of Surgery. pp. 390–420. New York, Brunner-Mazel 1976

10. **Jamison KR, Wellisch DK, Pasnau RO:** Psychosocial aspects of mastectomy I. The woman's perspective. Am J Psychiatry 135:432, 1978

11. **Wellisch DK, Jamison KR, Pasnau RO:** Psychosocial aspects of mastectomy II. The man's perspective. Am J Psychiatry 135:543, 1978

12. **Torrie A:** Like a bird with a broken wing. World Medicine 36, April, 1978

LEGAL IMPLICATIONS OF BREAST SURGERY

DENNIS M. MAHONEY

Because of the far-reaching legal ramifications of the plastic surgeon's venture into the field of super-elective surgery, it is necessary for the plastic surgeon who undertakes breast surgery to understand the legal implications involved.

Any understanding of the doctrine of informed consent must begin with a background detailing the earliest recorded thinking in this area. It is certainly clear that volumes of misinformation have been written concerning the doctrine of informed consent. It is likewise true that, to paraphrase Judge Learned Hand, physicians may actually feel that the doctrine of informed consent is the most horrific when on the fair face of justice.

It is my hope that, after reading this section and contemplating its ramifications, the physician community will perhaps have a more tolerant, if not kinder, opinion of the doctrine.

In 1914, Justice Cardozo iterated the then primordial beginnings of this legal doctrine. He said that "Every human being of adult years and sound mind has a right to determine what shall be done with his own body, and a surgeon who performs an operation without consent, commits an assault for which he is liable in damages.[5]

In 1928, Justice Brandeis phrased his thoughts in a somewhat different fashion as follows: "The makers of our constitution . . . sought to protect Americans in their beliefs, their thoughts, their emotions and their sensations. They conferred the right to be let alone—the most comprehensive of rights and the most valued by civilized men."[4] It would appear that Justice Brandeis in his thinking elevated the still unnamed concept of informed consent to its highest pinnacle—that of a constitutionally protected right.

Against the background of comments such as these from the most distinguished scholars of the legal profession, the doctrine of informed consent did not take shape until the 1960s. Prior to that time, cases sounding in consent were brought on the theory that the physician (surgeon) committed a battery upon the patient; that is, the doctrine generally encompassed situations in which a physician agreed with his patient to perform a particular operation, and at the time of surgery he either performed a different one or greatly exceeded the planned procedure. Hence the legal tort attached to such a set of circumstances was synonymous with the common-law concept of assault and battery.

In the 1960s, beginning with a case in Kansas,[2] courts began to inquire about the collateral risks and hazards of surgery with reference to information given to patients. Consent was not informed if, in fact, the patient was not told of the collateral risks and hazards of the surgery. In other words, in this type of situation, the patient only agreed to have a certain surgical procedure performed upon his body and precisely that procedure was to be performed. However, there is always a certain collateral risk inherent in surgery, and when that risk came to realization, the patient was injured. During the 1960s and into the early 1970s, the so-called doctrine of informed consent was utilized by a variety of courts. On each occasion, the court would indicate in its decision that the duty of the physician to disclose information was measured by, and consonant with, the degree of information being given to similar patients by physicians in the same or other medical communities. Hence, the duty to disclose and its parameters were measured by a physician standard of practice.

The natural corollary to this limitation was simply that expert medical testimony by physicians was a prerequisite for a patient to recover damages against a physician. In other words, if a physician was sued under the doctrine of lack of informed consent, the patient-plaintiff needed to produce a physician to testify under oath that, in fact, at the time and place in question the standard of surgical practice required the giving of information with reference to certain collateral risks and hazards. The physician would then list those particular collateral risks and hazards. This testimony, therefore, created the standard upon which the physician's conduct was to be judged. Without testimony from a physician detailing the above information, the plaintiff's case would not go to the jury and the suit would be dismissed. In legal terminology, the plaintiff had failed to establish a **prima facie** case of lack of informed consent.

In 1972, the most significant case in the history of the informed consent doctrine hit the medical and legal professions.[1] Judge Spottswood W. Robinson III wiped out the need for expert witness testimony on behalf of the plaintiff in an informed consent case.

Because this case radically changed the entire concept of informed consent, some background analysis would seem appropriate. The patient-plaintiff in this case was Mr. Canterbury, a 19-year-old clerk-typist, who was employed by the Federal Bureau of Investigation. In December of 1958 he began to develop severe pain between his shoulder blades. He was seen by several general practitioners and placed on medication, but the drugs failed to relieve the pain. Subsequently, he was seen by Dr. Spence, a neurosurgeon. Dr. Spence examined the plaintiff and found nothing of consequence during the clinical examination. Routine x-rays revealed no abnormality, but a myelogram revealed a filling defect in the region of the fourth thoracic vertebra. Dr. Spence told the plaintiff that he would have to undergo a laminectomy to correct what he suspected was a ruptured disk. The patient explained to Dr. Spence that his mother was a widow of thin financial means and that she could be reached by a neighbor's telephone in another state. After the myelogram, but before the proposed surgical procedure, the plaintiff's mother called Dr. Spence. Dr. Spence indicated that the surgery was occasioned by a suspected ruptured disk. Mrs. Canterbury then asked if the recommended operation was serious and Dr. Spence replied "Not any more than any other operation." The neurosurgeon indicated that he knew that Mrs. Canterbury was not well off financially and that her presence in Washington, D.C., would not be necessary.

The patient's mother did travel to Washington, D.C., and arrived on the day of the surgery but after the operative procedure was over. She signed a consent form on behalf of her son.

At the time of surgery, some anomalies of the spinal cord were found but, evidently, no ruptured disk. In the immediate postoperative period, the patient seemed to do well but then suffered a fall and ended up as a paraparetic with urinary incontinence and paralysis of the gastrointestinal tract.

Judge Robinson in his opinion began by discussing the background of the informed consent doctrine. Interestingly enough, he began his opinion by quoting Justice Cardozo. Judge Robinson continued in the opinion, explaining the nature of the physician-patient relationship and the fact that the partnership begins with, and is built upon, faith and trust. At page 782 of the opinion, it would appear that Judge Robinson elevates the physician-patient relationship to one of fiduciary with the following language: "More recently we ourselves have found in the fiducial qualities of the physician-patient relationship the physician's duty to reveal to the patient that which in his best interest it is important that he should know."

The court then discussed whether or not the traditional requirement of expert testimony was required in an informed consent case. Judge Robinson said "There are, in our view, formidable obstacles to acceptance of the notion that the physician's obligation to disclose is either germinated or limited by medical practice. To begin with, the reality of any discernable custom reflecting a professional consensus on communication of option and risk information to patients is open to serious doubt. We sense the danger that what, in fact, is no custom at all may be taken as an affirmative custom to maintain silence, and that physician-witnesses to the so-called custom may state merely their personal opinions as to what they or others would do under given conditions."

Judge Robinson concluded that there was no basis for operation of a special medical standard where the physician's conduct does not bring his medical knowledge and skills peculiarly into play. It is therefore axiomatic that where the challenge to the physician's conduct is not to be gauged by the special standard, medical custom cannot furnish the test of reasonable propriety.

Since **Canterbury vs. Spence** is clearly the trend of the law, it is important that physicians understand precisely its message. It is simply that the scope of the physician's communications to the patient must be measured by the patient's need to know. The patient must have the information required to make an appropriate decision whether or not to undergo surgery. All risks which potentially affect the decision of the patient must be uncovered. In order to safeguard the patient's interests in achieving and exercising his unbridled right to decide what is done with his body, the law must itself set the standard for adequate disclosure.

After analyzing the background standard against which the degree of information or lack thereof would be judged, the court turned to the question of subjective versus objective standard; that is, would the court allow the so-called subjective response of the injured plaintiff to the effect that "Had I known of this particular risk I would not have had surgery," or would the court indicate that the patient's retrospective self-serving response would be irrelevant. If the court were to follow the latter approach, then the only question would be whether or not a reasonable person standing in the position of the plaintiff would have required this or these pieces of information as prerequisites for an informed understanding of the procedure and its attendant risks and hazards. With relative unanimity, the jurisdictions adopting the **Canterbury** concept have thrown out the subjective interpretation and utilized the so-called objective reasonable man test.

In summary, the modern rule and clearly the trend of the law in the informed consent field is consonant with the **Canterbury vs. Spence** decision.

What are the ramifications of this decision to the daily private practice of plastic surgery? I am quick to point out to physicians that, in fact, there is no longer a debate as to whether or not a patient must receive an informed consent. The law is clear to the effect that patients must be told, and the breadth of the discussion is circumscribed by the patient's need to know, such that an intelligent decision can be made. No longer are discussions with reference to the morality or advisability of informed consent doctrines meaningful. It is the law. When a certain operation has a percentage risk of death or serious disability attendant to it, and the physician either knows of the risk or should know of the risk from the literature, he must indicate this information to that patient regardless of what other physicians in the same or similar communities are doing.

At this juncture, the plastic surgeon may wonder whether the doctrine has any salutary effect in his relationship with his patients. Those of us who deal with this concept on a daily basis are certainly of the consensus, if not the unanimous opinion, that the informed consent doctrine helps establish a meaningful physician-patient relationship. That is, we see again and again lawsuits beginning as a

result of unexpected injury. As an example, let's imagine a woman in her mid-30s with a seventh grade education. Her neighbor friend has had a cholecystectomy performed one year previously with no attendant problems or complications. Our patient finds out that she has gallstones and is going to require a cholecystectomy also. She only knows that her next-door neighbor had the same operation with no problems whatsoever. She asks her physician whether or not there are any risks in the operation and he promptly tells her that it's a safe and simple operation, that she will be hospitalized for a week and back at work in four weeks.

With this background information, she enters the hospital for her surgery. At the time of surgery, the physician lacerates the common bile duct and the liver. Both are successfully repaired but the common bile duct, of course, requires a stint. In the postoperative phase, the patient develops an ileus. After the ileus is controlled, the patient develops a subdiaphragmatic abscess, and this subdiaphragmatic abscess requires a second operative procedure to drain it. Subsequent to this second operation, the patient's wound dehisces. On top of these problems, the patient develops a pulmonary embolus and a superficial upper extremity phlebothrombosis from the continuing intravenous sites. Three months later, after approximately $46,000.00 worth of medical expense and lost wages and 40 pounds of weight loss, our hypothetical patient returns home. Can any physician in good conscience blame that hypothetical patient for filing a lawsuit against the surgeon based upon a lack of informed consent when the only information given her was both ill-advised and erroneous? Obviously not.

The significant impact of obtaining an informed consent from a patient is simply nothing more than having a forthright and candid discussion with the patient prior to surgery or any other operative diagnostic technique. If a patient believes that a physician has been candid and forthright in preoperative discussions, that same patient is less likely to seek legal help to file a subsequent medical malpractice claim. I am not unmindful of the Michigan study which has indicated that patients either forget or repress much of the medical data which is given to them preoperatively. That comes as no great surprise to the author. That study places in undeniable perspective the need for information in a written or other permanent form. It really matters little what the patient says he or she was told if, in fact, there is a detailed explanatory document or film which explains the operation and its attendant risks and hazards in lay language. The only question for determination as a threshold issue is whether or not the document actually contains the patient's signature or, in the case of a film, whether or not the catalogue information contains the patient's signature. Other inquiries such as whether or not the patient understood the information or slept through the information, etc., raise no particularly difficult or thorny legal or factual issues.

Statistics and background data are somewhat incomplete in terms of the actual role of the informed consent doctrine in medical malpractice verdicts or settlements. From our experience, it would seem that in at least 80 per cent of our medical malpractice cases the informed consent issue is raised if there has been a surgical procedure. It is true that the informed consent question is generally piggybacked with the so-called traditional theory of negligence. Cases in which the issue of informed consent is the sole cause of action sent to the jury for their consideration are relatively few. There have been, however, significant verdicts in both California and Ohio solely on the informed consent question. It is my view that, given the right circumstances—that is, a purely elective operative procedure, a clearly delineated and discernible risk which admittedly was not given to the patient, and a catastrophic injury—an award for a half million or a million dollars would not be out of the question.

What, then, should the plastic surgeon do prior to embarking on what I call super-elective (cosmetic) surgical procedures? He obviously must give the patient and the patient's husband or wife as much time as is necessary to explain precisely what he is going to do and what the significant collateral risks and hazards attendant to the operative procedure are, including general anesthetic risk if a general anesthetic is to be used. Next, such information must be given in a form capable of being preserved. Recently, we have advocated the use of films individualized for each elective operative event. Such film would be individualized for the particular procedure (i.e., augmentation mammaplasty, reduction mammaplasty, or facelift) and shown to the patient well in advance of the planned elective procedure. The film would be shown at a time when the patient is neither fiancially, emotionally, or psychologically geared to the operation. That is, the information should be given to the patient prior to the time that the patient's mother or father travels from a long distance to take care of the patient's children or otherwise help during the hospitalization. Such a financial and psychological constraint upon the patient, in my opinion, would be undue duress. Its net effect could only achieve an affirmative decision indicating the go-ahead for the surgery. All articles on this subject have discussed the need for a clear, nonsedated, and comprehensive intellect as a predicate to making the initial decision. I think it is important to point out that the physician need not give the information to the patient in a face-to-face or one-to-one presentation. The law only requires that the information be given, that it be given at a time when the patient has all of his or her options open, and that the information be truthful and accurate. Hence, it is our belief that films developed by specialists in the field who are acquainted with the literature make sense. We advocate a film of somewhere between 13 and 18 minutes in length. The film should not be a sales gimmick, but rather a truthful analysis of risks and hazards, including a reasonably anticipated range of results. Comments such as "You will not have scars" and "I will make you look like new" obviously are foolish and ill-advised. Such films can be shown to the patient in the physician's office, and a tear-off slip can be attached to the patient's chart indicating that on a particular date the patient has viewed the film.

A booklet reiterating the highlights of the film can be given to the patient to take home subsequent to the showing of the film, and there can be a place at the bottom of the handout for patient questions in response to the film. We like this particular format because we can not only preserve the film for showing to the judge and jury at the time of a possible later trial, but because we also feel such a film is useful at the outset in discouraging plaintiffs' medical malpractice cases prior to their filing. That is, if a patient seeks legal advice indicating that he or she was not informed of the risks and hazards of a particular operation, and the plaintiff's attorney views such a film, it is our belief that the vast majority of competent legal counsel will realize that they have little or no chance of prevailing on the consent issue. It is our belief, therefore, that many malpractice suits would not be filed. We are not naive enough to believe that such a procedure would obviate the filing of all medical malpractice suits. There will always be those among us, both lawyers and patients, who for one reason or another persist in the face of overwhelming evidence. It does seem clear, however, that the plaintiff's bar, while working on a contingency-fee basis, have more to do with their time than litigate cases which appear to be clearly in the losing category.

I should make clear that I am not so concerned about the particular magic of any one consent form or other document. I am more concerned that the document be truthful, that it incorporate substantial risks attendant to a procedure, and that the information given clearly antedates the time when financial and psychological constraints become operative.

If patients are told of the risk of death (anesthetic or otherwise) and the risk of serious bodily disability, it seems ludicrous to me to believe that a jury of reasonable men and women would or should conclude that this plaintiff was willing to accept such risks and not the risk of some excess scarring or loss of an implant. I view the problem of physician concern over the lack of incorporation of relatively minor risks in a consent form as a make-shift production of the physician community used solely to rationalize either indifference or inattentiveness. Many physicians immediately respond in informed consent discussions that "I don't have the time to teach a patient everything he or she needs to know. It took me 15 years of training to learn all that information." Such physicians do not understand the basic concept or the reasons behind it. No court of law has ever stated, nor will one ever state, that, in fact, any physician prior to surgery must teach a patient all there is to know about the operation and the hazards and risks attendant to it. It is clear that a patient must have reasonable information available so that he or she can determine whether the potential benefits to be derived from the operative procedure outweigh its attendant risks and hazards. Hence the importance of the information relative to death and serious bodily disability.

Many physicians actually believe that they know best what should be done for patients in the area of information supplied prior to elective surgery. In the law, this concept is rather euphemistically called the **parens patria** doctrine, which comes from the Latin concept of "parents know best." In Anglo-Saxon jurisprudence, the concept is utilized to mean that the state knows what is best for certain individuals (i.e., minors and those who are mentally incompetent). Lest some physicians believe that I relate this information tongue in cheek, I would refer them to a bill formulated by the New York Medical Society which actually codified this doctrine. The bill actually contained this language: "The medical practitioner, after considering all of the attendant facts and circumstances, used reasonable discretion as to the manner and extent to which such alternatives or risks were disclosed to the patient because he (physician) reasonably believed that the manner and extent of such disclosure could reasonably be expected to adversely and substantially affect the patient's condition.[3] If, in fact, the physician reasonably believed the above, his failure to give information would be a defense to a medical malpractice action based upon an informed consent theory.

It is my view that this particular section of such law is simply nothing more than a blatant codification of the **parens patriae** doctrine. Apart from the basic foolishness of such a concept in the informed consent field, it is my view that legislation such as this is totally counterproductive to the physician's best interests. If, as Judge Robinson says, the physician-patient experience is founded upon and buttressed by some sort of a fiduciary relationship, then the highest level of trust and free exchange of ideas must be utilized. It is my firm belief that Judge Robinson was correct in his thinking and that potential laws such as the one I have just discussed only serve to take the physician community a giant step backward in this most respected of all possible human relationships.

REFERENCES

1. Canterbury vs Spence, 464 F2d 772 (1972)
2. Natanson vs Kline, 186 Kan 393, 350 P2d 1093 (1963)
3. New York Public Health Law, §2805-D
4. Olmstead vs United States, 277 US 438, 478 (1928)

index

Numeral followed by an f indicates a figure; t following a numeral indicates tabular material.